THE YIN YOGA KIT
The Practice of Quiet Power

THE YIN YOGA KIT

The Practice of Quiet Power

BIFF MITHOEFER

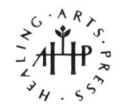

Healing Arts Press
Rochester, Vermont

Healing Arts Press
One Park Street
Rochester, Vermont 05767
www.HealingArtsPress.com

Healing Arts Press is a division of Inner Traditions International

Copyright © 2006 by Biff Mithoefer

All rights reserved. No part of this book may be reproduced or utilized in any form or by any means, electronic or mechanical, including photocopying, recording, or by any information storage and retrieval system, without permission in writing from the publisher.

Note to the reader: This book is intended as an informational guide. The remedies, approaches, and techniques described herein are meant to supplement, and not to be a substitute for, professional medical care or treatment. They should not be used to treat a serious ailment without prior consultation with a qualified health care professional.

Library of Congress Cataloging-in-Publication Data
Mithoefer, Biff.
 The yin yoga kit : the practice of quiet power / Biff Mithoefer.
   p. cm.
 ISBN-13: 978-1-59477-116-3
 1. Yin yoga. I. Title.
 RA781.73.M58 2006
 613.7'046—dc22

2006006906

Printed in China

10 9 8 7 6

Text design and layout by Priscilla Baker and Rachel Goldenberg
This book was typeset in Sabon with Perpetua Titling and Weiss as display typefaces
Interior photographs in Part 2 and the appendices by Rocki Pedersen

To send correspondence to the author of this book, mail a first-class letter to the author c/o Inner Traditions • Bear & Company, One Park Street, Rochester, VT 05767, and we will forward the communication.

CONTENTS

PREFACE

INTRODUCTION: THE PRACTICE OF YIN YOGA

Part 1
The Principles of Yin Yoga

YIN AND YANG	4
The Balance of Yin and Yang	6
QI	8
The Birth of Qi	8
Physical Qi	9
Resonance, Intention, Transformation, and Attachment	10
Encouraging the Flow of Qi	12
THE TAOIST MERIDIAN SYSTEM	13
Table: Meridian Attributes	18

THE TANTRIC CHAKRA SYSTEM	19
Table: Chakra Attributes	28
YIN POSTURES, MERIDIANS, AND ENERGY CENTERS	29
Table: Meridians and Energy Centers Affected by Each Yin Posture	30

Part 2
Practicing Yin Yoga

GUIDELINES FOR A YIN YOGA PRACTICE	32
THE YIN YOGA POSTURES	34
Resting Pose	37
Half Butterfly	40
Butterfly	43
Square Pose	45
Shoelace	47
Seal	49
Saddle	52
Swan	55
Sleeping Swan	58
Forward Bend	60
Dragonfly	63
Frog	65
Spinal Twist	67
Final Relaxation	69
THE PRACTICE OF MINDFULNESS	71
THE PRACTICE OF LOVING KINDNESS	76

USING THE YIN YOGA KIT	
TO DESIGN YOUR PERSONAL PRACTICE	79
How to Use the Yin Yoga CD	79
How to Use the Yin Yoga Cards	82
The Use of Props	85

Part 3
Anatomy and Yin Yoga

THE CONNECTIVE TISSUE	88
THE SACRUM AND THE LUMBAR SPINE	91
Relaxing the Iliopsoas	92
TENSION AND COMPRESSION	95
MOVEMENT IN THE HIPS AND SPINE	101
Movement in the Hip Joints	101
Movement in the Spine	103
Table: Spine and Hip Movements in Yin Postures	108
APPENDIX 1: SOME SAMPLE PRACTICES	109
APPENDIX 2: PRACTICES FOR SPECIFIC ORGAN MERIDIANS	117
APPENDIX 3: USING ACUPRESSURE POINTS	
WHILE PRACTICING YIN YOGA	122
RESOURCES	128
ACKNOWLEDGMENTS	130

*So let the body speak for you now
without you saying a word,
like the student walking
behind the teacher says
this one knows better than I the way.*
					RUMI

PREFACE

The path of Yin Yoga has its foundation in ancient yogic and Taoist (Daoist) theory. The modern practice was first developed by Paul Grilley, drawing on these ancient teachings. Paul's theories grew from his own knowledge of the human body and from his teachers, Pulie Zink and Dr. Hiroshi Motoyama. The form of Yin Yoga that I have presented here has its roots in the understanding I've gained from my teachers—Paul Grilley, Sarah Powers, and Don and Amba Stapleton. My deepest teachings, however, have come from my own practice and from that well of knowledge that each of us has available inside ourselves—the wisdom of our own bodies. Like all spiritual practices, Yin Yoga asks us to seek our own truths and to accept the teachings of others only when those teachings feel true to us. With this in mind, I suggest that you take this practice as it comes to you and make it your own.

INTRODUCTION: THE PRACTICE OF YIN YOGA

The practice of Yin Yoga addresses the more yin parts of the body. These are the parts of ourselves that lie closest to our core, specifically the bones and connective tissue above the knees and below the navel. Unlike the muscles, which are the more yang parts of our bodies—the parts that like movement and repetition—the connective tissue needs to be addressed in a yin way with an attitude of quiet acceptance. The postures are all practiced on the floor and each is held for a long period, usually three to five minutes. By putting ourselves in safe and controlled positions, we can relax the muscles around the areas we're working, allowing the connective tissue to be gently and safely maintained.

Because yin doesn't exist without yang, yin practice also affects the yang tissues of the body, stretching and strengthening the muscles. But because of the way Yin Yoga is practiced, its primary affect is on the more yin tissue. Yin Yoga is not a replacement for more yang forms of yoga or exercise, but a complement to them, helping to bring balance in our lives.

For me, the practice of Yin Yoga is important for four reasons:

1. It helps balance the yin and yang aspects of ourselves.
2. It encourages the increased flow of qi or prana, primarily in the six meridians of the body that pass through the area of the hips.
3. It helps to maintain the health of the connective tissue.
4. It helps us develop a mindful meditation practice.

In Part 1 of this book you can read more about the principles underlying these Yin Yoga benefits—the Taoist concept of yin and yang, the life energy known as *qi* or *prana,* the Taoist meridian system of energy flow, and the tantric chakra system of energy concentration.

Part 2 presents the actual practice of Yin Yoga, including illustrated instructions for each of the fourteen postures in the basic practice, as well as an introduction to the practices of mindfulness and loving kindness that for me are at the heart of Yin Yoga. Part 2 will also help you use the materials in the *Yin Yoga Kit* to design your own personal practice. It will tell you how to use the audio CD and the posture cards included in the kit, offer some advice on the use of props, and give you guidance on how to choose a sequence of postures that will meet your needs at any given time.

Part 3 focuses on the intersection of Yin Yoga and human anatomy. It shows how the practice revitalizes the connective tissue and restores the natural curve of the sacrum and lumbar spine; explains the ways that tension and compression restrict range of motion; discusses the natural range of movement in the hips and the spine; and gives recognition to the fact that individual physical differences will make each person's practice unique.

Along with information on combining accupressure with Yin Yoga, the appendices present several sample practice sequences to help you get started, but it is my hope that you will use the information and materials offered here to design the perfect practice for you.

Part 1

The Principles of Yin Yoga

YIN AND YANG

The word *yoga* in Sanskrit means "to yoke" or "to bind together" and refers to the bringing together or balancing of two opposing forces. In hatha yoga, these forces are represented by the Sanskrit words *ha,* meaning "sun," and *tha,* meaning "moon." In the Taoist tradition of China, the words *yang* and *yin* are used to hold the two sides of this same paradox. In the context of Yin Yoga, I'll use the terms *yin* and *yang* when discussing these ideas.

Yin and *yang* are terms of relativity. Something is only yin or yang in relation to something else, so the concepts of yin and yang are about relationship. The word *yin* literally means "the shady side of the mountain," while *yang* means "the sunny side of the mountain."

All that we know—the universe, our bodies, our emotions, our thoughts, our spiritual selves—is always in a state of balance or imbalance between these two forces. The yang side of our nature, our emotions, our spirit, our world, is that part that is most active, most upwardly focused, warmer, closer to the surface, most fluid, most focused on change and striving, most masculine. It's this yang part of us that sees the world and ourselves in terms of how things should be different, how we need to change things to make them more the way we think they ought to be. The yin side of the natural world and of ourselves is less active, cooler, closer to the core, more earth oriented, dryer, more receptive, more at peace with how things are, more feminine. It is our yin self that holds our compassionate, accepting mother energy. Physically, some of our more yang parts are our skin and muscles, the parts that thrive on movement and change, whereas our yin parts are our bones and deep connective tissue, which are more stable and change only slowly.

All that is manifested—the things we see, the things we think we know, our thoughts, our emotions, all that we can perceive with our mind—is made up of yin and yang. And anything we perceive as being either yin or yang can be broken down further into it's own yin and yang aspects. Let's take look at movement, for example: since slow movement is more yin and faster movement is more yang, walking would be considered yin in relationship to running, which is more yang. But if we break it down further, we can see that slow walking would be considered yang when compared to even slower crawling. In the paradigm of yin and yang, there are no absolutes.

Yin and yang exist only because of each other. They co-create each other. Without fast there would be no slow. As Lao Tsu says: "Under heaven all can see beauty only because there is ugliness."

When we can truly understand this idea, we can begin to drop the assumptions we hold about what is good and what is bad; we can begin to embrace all that comes to us without judgment. When we see clearly that our sadness is a necessary part of our joy and that, in fact, they create each other, we can loosen the bindings that attach us so strongly to the way we think things should be.

Not only do yin and yang create each other; once created, they control each other. If you move slowly, in a yin way, then there will be an absence of speed or yang nature. As we move more slowly, we also move less quickly.

Yin and yang are in a constant state of transformation, yin becoming yang and yang becoming yin. Understanding this, we know that as night becomes day and winter becomes summer, our sufferings become joy, our anger becomes peace, and our hate becomes love. It is only the clinging of our minds that makes us forget, that makes us see impermanence as permanence. By understanding that yin and yang, even in their duality, are but two sides of the same mountain, we can begin to understand that we can never be separate from one another, from nature, or from our true selves.

The Balance of Yin and Yang

Much of our physical, emotional, and spiritual health depends on the balance of yin and yang in ourselves. In a global context, this balance is also crucial for the health and survival of our planet. Taoist tradition says that when we are in balance we live in accordance with the flow of life, the Tao (Dao).

We hold within ourselves a paradox. We all have a yang nature, the part of ourselves that needs change, that needs to strive to make things the way we think they should be. This is a necessary part of life. We also hold a yin nature, the part that is accepting, that knows that everything is really all right just the way it is.

I believe that for many of us, and for the world in general, the yang side has become dominant. We live in a world where we are often told that we're not good enough, that things aren't right the way they are. It often feels like a world where striving has become more important than accepting.

The practice of Yin Yoga can help us understand the value of acceptance at a deep cellular level. By holding postures without trying to change things, by just accepting ourselves as we are, we can begin to feel the yin parts of ourselves. Needing for things to be different than how they are brings us to a place of judgment and blame and takes us out of ourselves and out of the perfect present moment.

I believe that it's time for us to reclaim our yin nature, both for our own health and for the health of our planet. We ache in our hearts for the nurturing comfort of the Goddess.

> *You do not have to walk on your knees*
> *For a hundred miles through the desert repenting.*
> *You only have to let the soft animal of your body*
> *Love what it loves.*
>
> MARY OLIVER,
FROM "WILD GEESE"

QI

Along with the concept of yin and yang, qi (pronounced chi) lies at the core of the Taoist view of the cosmos. Qi is often referred to as the life force but it is really much more than that. Just as yin and yang can't be separated from each other, qi as energy can't be separated from qi as matter. Modern quantum physics defines light as neither particle nor wave but as more of a wave of possibility. Qi is like that wave of possibility. It is neither energy nor matter; it is the potential of both. Like the transformation of yin to yang and yang to yin, qi is the transformation of energy to matter and matter to energy. Embracing and including both, but in fact being neither, qi is the energy that caused the big bang and at the same time it is all that has been manifested from it.

The Birth of Qi

In Taoist cosmology, the source of qi is the Tao, which is the mystery behind everything, the way, the natural unfolding of the cosmos. It is that which can't be named but whose presence we sense in our hearts.

The poet Rumi refers to it when he says,

This that we have now is not imagination
It is not joy or sadness
Not grief or elation
These things come and go
This is the presence that doesn't.

From this eternal mystery called the Tao, comes the birth of qi and from it the manifestation of all things. For Taoists, all phenomena, including our physical bodies, the natural world, and even our thoughts and emotions, follow this threefold path of existence. The Tao is considered to be the essence, the true nature, and the potential of everything. It is the natural order of the cosmos, the reason that all in nature exists. From the Tao, qi arises. This qi is the subtle energy that manifests the potential of the Tao. These three stages—the Tao, qi, and all manifested phenomena—are not really stages at all but are holistic concepts. The Tao is not separate from qi or manifested phenomena; it includes them. All matter contains qi, as well as the potential or essence that is the Tao. It is only our way of seeing things and speaking about things that make us separate one thing from another to create duality. Taoism, in its nonduality, is very hard to speak of, but as we practice we can begin to understand it at a deeper more essential level.

Physical Qi

While qi in its unmanifested form represents the mystery that like the Tao is unnamable, in its manifested form we speak of qi as being present in our bodies. In this form we think of it as being more like energy. It is this qi flowing within our bodies that gives us life. Whereas qi in its universal, unmanifested form is both yin and yang, in its more physical form it is thought of it in terms of its yang nature—its ability to bring movement, warmth, stability, and health to the body. Qi is present in, and necessary to, the transformations that constantly take place within us.

On a physical level, qi enters the body in three forms:

Prenatal Qi, or that which we bring into this world with us from our ancestors;
Grain Qi, which we get from the food we eat; and
Natural Air Qi, which we gather from the air we breathe.

In the Taoist view, it is the free, smooth flow of this qi to all parts of the body (particularly to our major organs) that brings us physical and emotional health. When qi flows smoothly and strongly, we're healthy and our qi is said to be harmonious. When qi is in disharmony, it is classified under the broad categories of being either deficient or stagnant.

In its milder form, deficient qi doesn't allow us the energy to fully embrace life. We can feel tired, lazy, and unenthusiastic. In more severe cases of deficient qi, the organs lose their ability to function fully or even to be held in their proper places within the body. When qi becomes stagnant it loses its ability to flow where it's needed. Its flow is restricted or in some cases even reversed. Both stagnant and deficient qi are conditions of disharmony that affect the health of our organs and our whole body. Qi is like the water that brings life to a garden. If the hose that we use to water the garden is kinked (stagnant) or the faucet is only turned part way on (deficient), the plants will suffer from lack of life-giving moisture.

Resonance, Intention, Transformation, and Attachment

Qi is not an energy that causes change, although it is present during change. Qi is the magic that joins all things. It is through the mystery of qi that all things are connected. Through qi, our every word, action or thought affects all other manifested phenomenon. A physicist would describe this universal connection of all things with the theory of nonlocality. Change is transformation; things transform or change because they contain that into which they change. Qi is that connection, that common thread, between one form of existence and the next. In Taoist terms, change only occurs through resonance *(gan ying)*. A caterpillar contains the seed (qi) of a butterfly but for metamorphosis to occur there needs to be a resonance (gan ying) between that caterpillar and its butterflyness. When the weather begins to cool and the days grow shorter, the caterpillar begins to feel the change. A resonance between it and the butterfly, which it both is and will become, begins the transformation. In the same way, we contain many seeds of possibility. When we are sick, we also contain the seed of wellness. It is the job of the healer—whether an Oriental doctor or ourselves in our own yoga practice—not to try to force a change from sickness to wellness but to look for that which encourages the resonance between the two. In the same way, while recognizing that we contain joy and sadness, peace and violence, courage and fear, we need to find a practice or a way of life that will help us to water the seeds that bring us to our true heart's desire.

Intention is a way of actively bringing resonance to our lives. We often feel helpless to bring about the changes in ourselves and in our world that we think are needed. When we look deeply, we see that all we can really control is our intention. Understanding that the seed for change is always there, we know that our true intention is really all we need. Much of our suffering comes from thinking we can and must ultimately control the outcome of our intentions or our actions. This is called attachment to the results of our actions. We experience attachment when we are dominated by our yang nature. Of course, both our yin and yang natures want things to be better for ourselves and all beings, but it is our yang nature—our striving ego self—that really believes that the end result of our action is what's most important. When we open ourselves more to our accepting, compassionate yin nature, we can embrace our good, true intention and know that that's all we truly have to offer, all we can really control. And that it's enough.

Encouraging the Flow of Qi

In his book *The Healing Promise of Qi,* Dr. Roger Jahnke discusses an ancient qigong practice called the "Three Intentful Corrections" or "Three Focal Points." Dr. Jahnke suggests this practice as a good way to start encouraging the flow of qi. The three focal points are as follows:

- "Adjust and regulate the body posture"
- "Adjust and regulate the breath"
- "Adjust and regulate consciousness"

I have found that these same concepts form the basis of the five ways that I encourage the flow of qi in my own Yin Yoga practice.

1. By assuming a physical posture that brings gentle tension to parts of the body where the meridians can be easily affected
2. By bringing attention to the breath, which can include sending the breath to a particular part of the body
3. By opening my consciousness to the possibility of freeing the flow of qi, to the possibility of healing
   Once I have brought focus to these three areas I can then
4. Bring mental attention to
   - The specfic part of the body being affected by the posture
   - The meridians and their related organs most affected by the posture
   - The particular chakras most affected by the posture
5. Apply pressure to specific acupressure points

THE TAOIST MERIDIAN SYSTEM

In Taoist theory the human body is alive because of the mysterious life energy called qi. In hatha yoga this life force is known as prana. Qi flows throughout the body, bringing health and vitality to every cell. Although qi is present everywhere in the body, it flows mainly in certain pathways called meridians, which guide qi to specific parts of the body, most importantly to the vital organs. Taoists have identified fourteen meridians, twelve of which relate to the major organs of the body. The twelve organ meridians are the Lung, Large Intestine, Stomach, Spleen, Heart, Small Intestine, Urinary Bladder, Kidney, Gall Bladder, Liver, Pericardium, and Triple Heater meridians. It is the free flow of energy to the organs that keeps them healthy and functioning properly. When the qi in a meridian is blocked or slowed, the organ that corresponds to that meridian is affected and the whole body suffers. In the Taoist view, disease is only a symptom of some blockage or irregularity in the flow of qi.

The intention of all yoga, and Yin Yoga in particular, is to keep energy flowing smoothly throughout the body. In this Yin Yoga practice we focus on the six lower-body organ meridians, those that pass through the area of the hips: the Urinary Bladder, Stomach, Gall Bladder, Spleen, Liver, and Kidney meridians. Although the practice brings particular attention and healing to these lower-body meridians, it has a beneficial influence on the whole body because each of the lower-body meridians has a direct relationship with an upper-body meridian. The lower-body and upper-body meridians are paired as follows: Urinary Bladder/Small Intestine, Stomach/Large Intestine, Gall Bladder/Triple heater, Spleen/Lung, Liver/Pericardium, and Kidney/Heart.

The work of Dr. Hiroshi Motoyama, a Shinto priest and founder of the California Institute for Human Sciences, and others has helped confirm the existence of the meridians. It is understood by Dr. Motomoya and by many in the field of Oriental medicine that the majority of blockages to the free flow of qi occur within the dense connective tissue in the major joints of the body. Yin Yoga targets the connective tissue surrounding the lower back, the pelvis, and the joints of the femurs. By bringing our attention to these areas through mental or physical concentration, we can stimulate the flow of qi in much the same way that acupuncture does. (In Appendix 3, I suggest some acupuncture points that can be pressed while in Yin Yoga postures to bring added stimulus to the meridians.)

In this book and card set I've indicated which lower-body meridians seem most affected by particular Yin postures in my own experience and for those with whom I've practiced. As each person's body is different, you may feel the effects of a posture in a whole different way. *Please trust your own experience.*

In general, the deeper forward bends, such as Half Butterfly, Frog, Forward Bend, Dragonfly, and Square Pose stretch and affect the Urinary Bladder meridian, which runs down the backs of the legs. Postures such as Seal, Saddle, and Swan can also affect the Urinary Bladder meridian as a result of compression where it passes through the area of the lower back.

The Stomach meridian, which flows down the front (anterior) side of the thigh, passing through the outside (lateral) portion of the knee

Urinary Bladder meridian

Stomach meridian

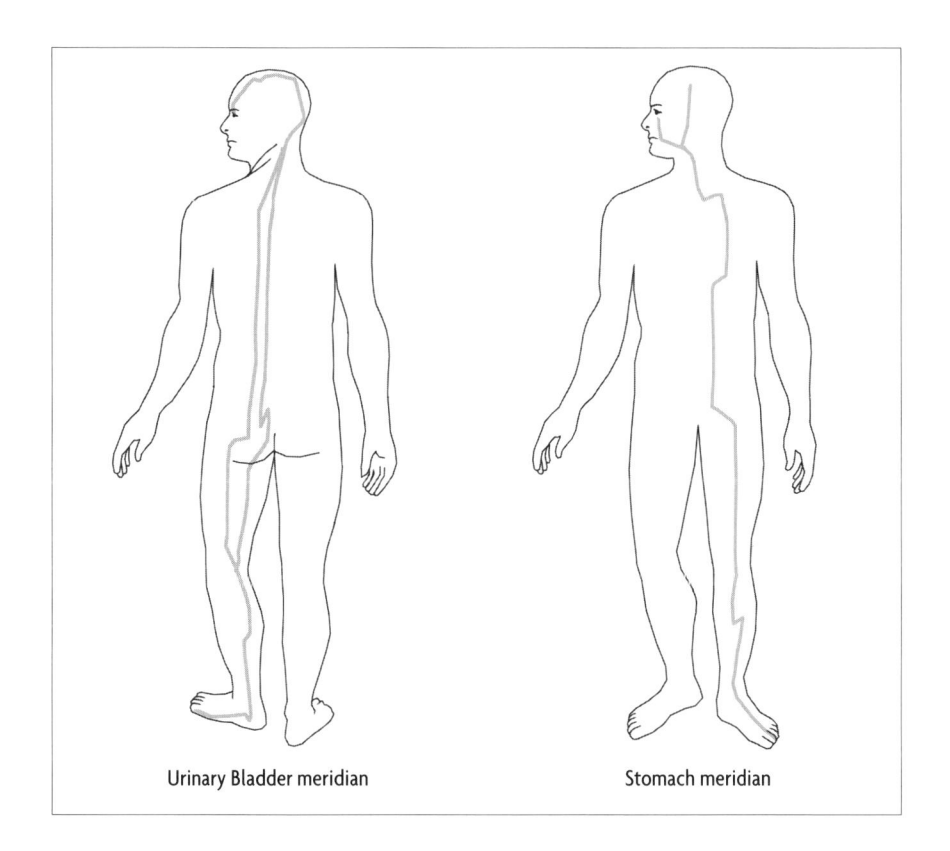

and continuing down the shin, is also influenced by Seal, Saddle, and Swan because of the stretch that these postures exert on that part of the legs.

The Gall Bladder meridian flows down the outsides of the legs after exiting the area of the abdomen. This meridian is often affected as we rotate the legs in relation to the torso. These rotations occur in Half Butterfly, Square Pose, Swan, Sleeping Swan, Spinal Twist, and Shoelace. For a few people, the Gall Bladder meridian can also be affected in Butterfly.

The Spleen meridian runs upward along the front inside (anterior medial) portion of the legs. It tends to be stimulated by stretching in the back bends, Seal, Saddle, and Swan. It's also stimulated by compression in Sleeping Swan, and for some people, in Frog.

Gall Bladder meridian

Spleen meridian

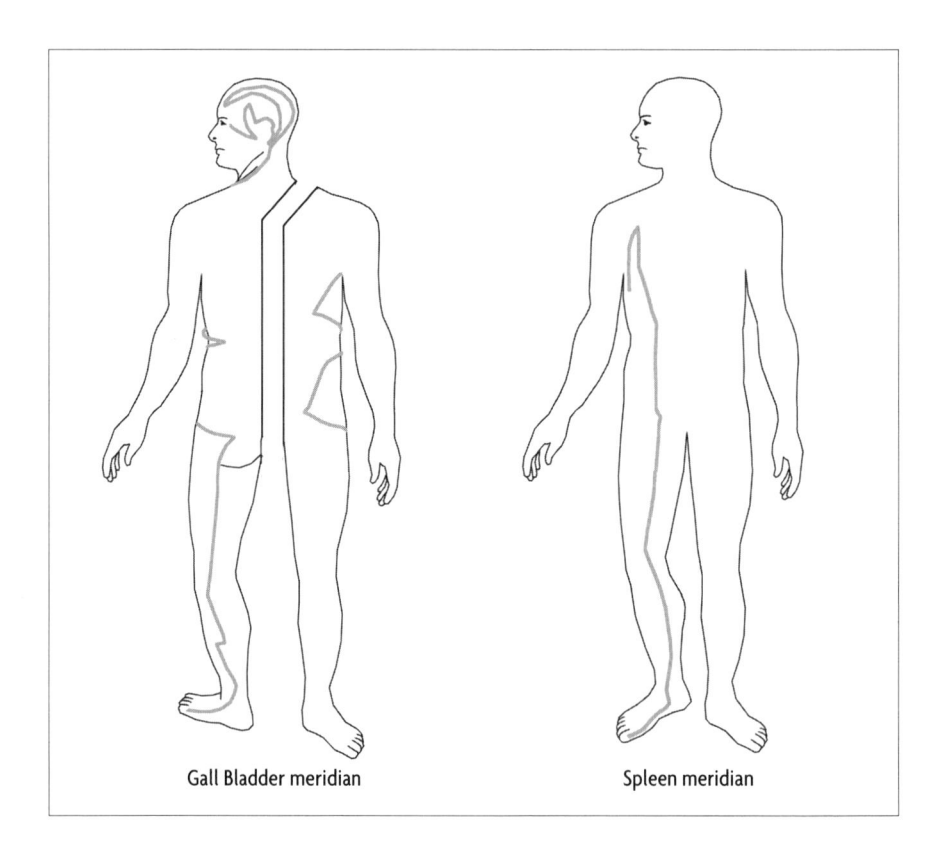

The Liver meridian ascends along the inside (medial) aspect of the legs before entering the body and progressing into the chest. The actual meridian ends in the chest but from there it energetically reconstitutes itself, following the trachea upward to the throat, with its influence ultimately reaching the top of the head. It's affected by stretching in postures in which the thigh bones (femurs) are abducted—spread open away from the midline of the body—such as Butterfly, Half Butterfly, Dragonfly, and Frog. Some people also feel the Liver meridian in Shoelace because their legs are rotated outward (externally rotated) and compressed by the forward bending of the posture. It is also possible to feel the effect of Spinal Twist on the Liver meridian.

The Kidney meridian, like the Liver meridian, runs up the insides of the legs and is generally affected by the same postures. When the Kidney

Liver meridian

Kidney meridian

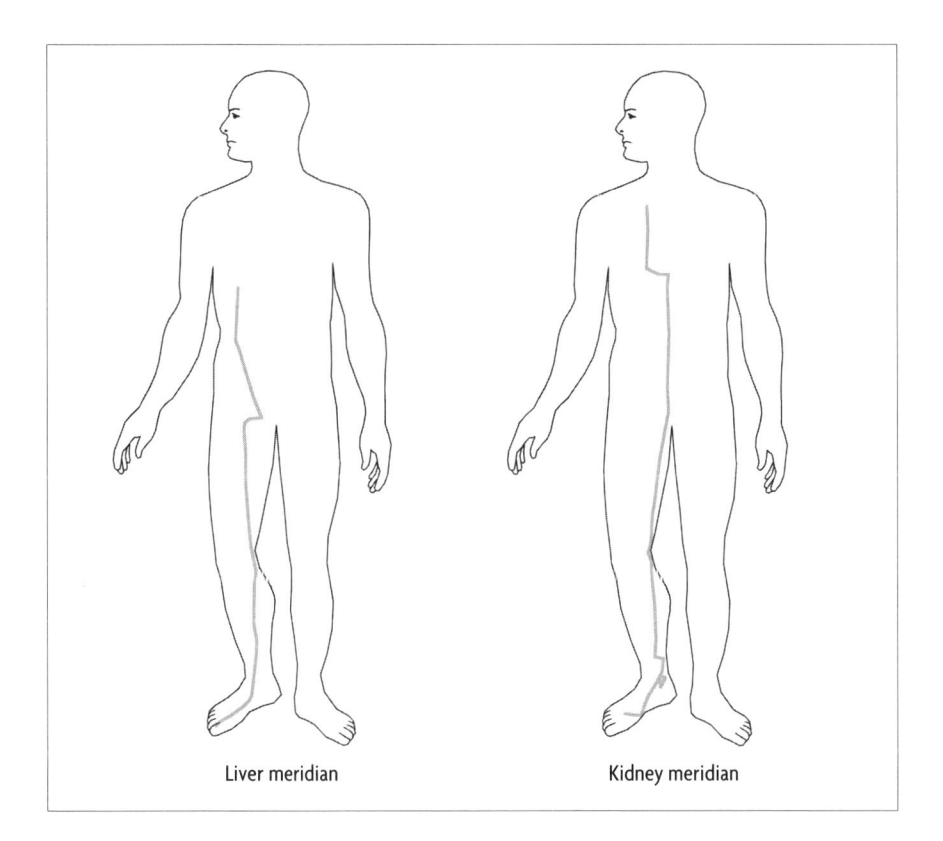

meridian enters the body near the base of the spine it passes very close to the coccyx, sacrum, and lumbar spine. In this area it's affected by the backbends: Seal, Swan, and particularly Saddle. As with the Liver meridian, some people will feel the effect of Spinal Twist on the Kidney meridian.

The Meridian Attributes table on the next page outlines the emotional attributes of each meridian as characterized by the Taoist or Oriental medical paradigm, as well as the classical emotional symptoms that can occur when the meridian is in disharmony. The table also includes the Yin Yoga postures that are most likely to stimulate certain meridians, as explained above. The last column of the table lists the chakras that are most often related to particular meridians. I will speak in more detail about the chakras in the next chapter.

MERIDIAN ATTRIBUTES

Meridian	Positive Attributes	Negative Attributes	Postures Stimulating	Related Chakras
Gall Bladder (Yang)	Courage, Decisiveness	Rash Decisions, Easily Frightened, Indecisive, Annoyed by Little Things	Half Butterfly, Square, Swans, Spinal Twist, Shoelace	3rd Chakra
Stomach (Yang)	Sympathy, Compassion	Explosive Behavior, Moodiness, Suspiciousness Paranoia, Nervousness, Readily Influenced by Others	Seal, Saddle, Swans	3rd Chakra
Urinary Bladder (Yang)	The Urinary Bladder meridian is closely related to the Kidney meridian and is strongly influenced by it	Disharmonies are most often physically manifested	Half Butterfly, Frog, Seal, Forward Bend, Dragonfly, Square, Swan, Saddle	1st and 2nd Chakra
Kidney (Yin)	Wisdom, Gentleness, Home of our Essence (Jing). Both yin and yang Will come from the Kidney	Fear, Dread of Death, Locked in Grief	Half Butterfly, Shoelace, Frog, Seal, Butterfly, Dragonfly, Swan, Saddle	1st and 2nd Chakra
Spleen (Yin)	Faithfulness, Source of Potentials, Possibilities, Motivations, Creativity	Pensiveness, Worry Easily, Trouble Making Decisions	Frog, Seal, Swans, Saddle	3rd Chakra
Liver (Yin)	The Seat of Human Kindness	Anger	Half Butterfly, Shoelace, Frog, Butterfly, Dragonfly	3rd Chakra

THE TANTRIC CHAKRA SYSTEM

The word *chakra*, or "wheel," in Sanskrit refers to the tantric system of energy centers that exist in the physical, emotional, and spiritual bodies. The chakras, like the meridians, represent places where energy is concentrated. The chakras, however, don't guide energy flow from one place to another in the body in quite the way the meridians do, but are more centers of energy in themselves. At each chakra the concentrated energy spins around a central point, like a wheel spinning around an axle. Different traditions have different views about the number and location of the chakras, but for our purposes I refer to seven chakras that lie along the length of the spine, from the first chakra at its base to the seventh chakra above the crown of the head.

Dr. Motoyama and others have shown a direct relationship between the Taoist meridian theory of China and the tantric chakra system of India. Each Yin Yoga posture affects not only one or more meridians, but their corresponding chakras as well. By understanding which chakras are most affected by a particular posture, we can bring our attention to them, promoting increased energy flow through their associated meridians and organs.

In the same way that the Taoist system views the energy in each meridian or organ as being in a state of harmony or disharmony, the chakra system evaluates the quality of energy within each chakra. When a particular chakra is functioning well, it is considered to be open in a healthy way. If it is malfunctioning, it is considered to be either blocked or excessively open.

The chakras are located in specific parts of the body where they affect, and are affected by, the nearby organs, nerves, and glands. Each chakra represents a different archetypal human characteristic. The archetype each represents is dependent not only on the placement of the chakra, but also on the quality of energy flow within it—that is, on whether the chakra is open with a sufficient flow of energy, blocked, or excessively open. Our emotional states are also considered to be closely related to the state of our chakras. With the exception of the seventh chakra, each chakra is associated with a different element and is seen as holding the energy of that element.

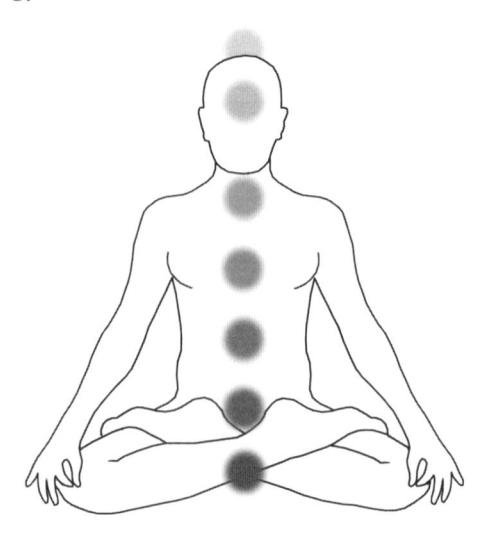

The seven chakras are located along the spine from the root chakra at its base to the crown chakra just above the crown of the head.

Yin Yoga primarily affects the first three chakras, although, of course, through the power of attention and intention, we can affect all aspects of ourselves, and therefore all of our chakras.

The first chakra, or Muladhara in Sanskrit, is also known as the root chakra. It is located at the base of the spine in the area of the coccyx. The issues associated with the first chakra have to do with our feeling of belonging on the earth and in our bodies. The element related to it is earth. When the first chakra is open, the archetype it helps us manifest is that of the Earth Mother. This is the part of our nature that holds the earth and all beings with compassion and caring. It is the part of ourselves that feels tied to the earth and to our bodies. When our Earth Mother self is present, we feel at home on the earth. We know that there is space for us and that we'll be taken care of, just as we take care of others and nature. When our first chakra is blocked, we are apt to manifest the negative archetype of the Victim. The Victim is that part of ourselves that feels that we're not getting our full share of attention and care. We can feel insecure or fearful, disassociated from our bodies and others. People who are blocked in their root chakras often feel that they aren't worthy of taking up space on Earth. An excessively open first chakra is likely to manifest as extreme materialism, running to greed and hoarding. The demon of Muladhara is fear. Its affirmation is "I have the right to be."

The second chakra is known as Svadhisthana in Sanskrit, which means, "to dwell with relish in one's own place." It is located in the area of the sacrum and genitals and is closely related to the hips and their movement. The second chakra is associated with our sexuality and all the issues that surround it. In our modern culture, with its confused messages and views on human sexuality, the second chakra is a place where many people feel closed or conflicted. The second chakra also deals with issues of pleasure and its companion, pain. By not accepting our right to find pleasure and joy in all aspects of ourselves, we leave ourselves open to the demon of the second chakra—guilt. When we live with the feeling that we don't deserve the happiness we experience, it is very easy to let guilt replace our joy. This is particularly true around issues of sexuality. People who are blocked in the second chakra are apt to be very rigid. They may be restricted emotionally, in their physical movement, and in their sexuality. When this chakra is excessively open, it may manifest as a person with weak boundaries, who has little discretion emotionally or sexually. Such a person often has an excessive need to be constantly connected with others. The archetype of the second chakra is the Lover. This is the Lover in a physical, passionate way, as opposed to the archetype of the heart chakra, which is more about compassion and healing. The negative archetype of this chakra, which manifests when second-chakra energy is blocked, is the Martyr, the person who takes satisfaction from denying his or her own pleasure and happiness. The element associated with Svadhisthana is water. At the second chakra, located in the area around the sacrum and hips, we have moved from the grounded stability of first chakra, rooted at the base of the spine, to a place of more movement and fluidity. The second chakra is about embracing movement and change in our lives. Whereas the first chakra is very much about ourselves and our need to feel secure, the second chakra begins to include our need to be with others. The affirmation of Svadhisthana is "I have the right to feel."

The third chakra, also known as Manipura, which means "lustrous gem" in Sanskrit, is located in the area of the solar plexus. This chakra is associated with our ego and our feelings of autonomy. It's about our personal power and our will. It is here that we learn to individuate. When the third chakra is open, it manifests feelings of self-confidence and self-esteem. The excessively open third chakra tends to manifest as a kind of willpower that is more inflexible than it is strong. People with excessive Manipura chakras are often aggressive in a bullying way, always needing to be in charge. Blockage in the third chakra may show up as selfless behavior that is motivated by shame and feelings of personal worthlessness, rather than by devotion. From the elements of earth and water in the first and second chakras, we move to the element of fire in the third. The archetype of Manipura is the Hero. The archetypal Hero is someone who leaves the security of his home and, with confidence, begins a journey to find his own treasure, his own way. The negative third-chakra archetype is the Servant or Slave. This is someone who doesn't have enough self-confidence to pursue his or her own journey, but can only follow the ways of others. Servants don't identify with themselves; they are concerned only with another's acceptance of them. The demon here is shame, the shame that keeps us from living as our true self desires. The affirmation of the third chakra is, "I have the right to act, the right to follow my path."

The fourth chakra, or Anahata in Sanskrit, which means, "the unstruck sound," is located at the heart. From the fire of the third chakra, we move into the element of air and the gentleness of the heart at the fourth chakra. The issues associated with it are love, compassion, balance, devotion, and selfless service. The fourth chakra deals with bringing balance and intimacy to relationships. When this chakra is open we can feel unconditional love—love without need or expectation. We can have true compassion for ourselves and for others. This is compassion without pity. When Anahata is excessively open, love can become codependent, with the emphasis being turned outward. Love can be used for its own purpose, with little room left for another. When the fourth chakra is blocked, love can become conditional. Or a person with fourth-chakra blockages may withdraw from love, fearful of being wounded, and live with a feeling of being unlovable. The archetype of the heart chakra is the Healer. As Angeles Arrien says, in her book *The Four-Fold Way: Walking the Paths of the Warrior, Teacher, Healer and Visionary,*

"The task of the healer is to pay attention to what has heart and meaning" and to access the "power of love." The negative archetype is the Actor. The actor doesn't really come from his or her own heart but uses acting skills to appear sincere. The demon of the fourth chakra is grief. Grief can cause us to withdraw from our own hearts. The affirmation of Anahata is, "I have the right to love and to be loved."

Although I believe that the fifth, sixth, and seventh chakras are not directly influenced by the Yin Yoga postures I've presented, they can be affected by our intentions in any posture, so I will briefly discuss them.

The fifth chakra, Vishuddha in Sanskrit, which means "pure," is located at the throat. Its issues are around communication and self-expression. When this chakra is open we can find our own voice, we feel able to speak our own truth. The fifth chakra relates to all kinds of self-expression, in speech and in other creative mediums. When Vishuddha is blocked, it can manifest as an inability to put words together, with attempts at communication churning back into oneself. People with blocked fifth chakras may be able to communicate about unimportant things, but unable to speak about what is really true for them. Some people may not be able to communicate at all. When Vishuddha is excessively open, one may talk constantly, using speech as a mechanism of control. The excessive speech functions as a defense and a way to avoid revealing real feelings. The archetype of the fifth chakra is the Communicator or Artist, the person who is comfortable with true self-expression. The negative archetype is the Silent Child. This is the part of ourselves that is afraid to speak, to express our own needs and truths. The demons of Vishuddha are lies. The fifth-chakra affirmation is "I have the right to speak and to be heard."

The sixth chakra, Ajna in Sanskrit, is also known as the third eye. It is located at the center of the forehead. Some of the issues of the sixth chakra are clarity, vision, insight, and imagination. When Ajna is open we can see things as they really are. We can remove the veils that we have allowed to cloud our vision. These veils or filters, through which we so often view life, are given to us by our families, our culture, and ourselves. I believe that they are also a part of what we enter this life with. This clarity of the sixth chakra can manifest at the physical level, allowing us to see what is really before us on the physical plane without the prejudices, positive or negative, that we often carry. As Anais Nin has written, "We don't see things as they are, we see things as we are." It is only when we are clear ourselves that we can see clearly. The sixth chakra can also open us to see clearly at the astral and causal planes. At these planes we develop imagination, insight, intuition, and clairvoyance. It's through the opening of the third eye that we are able see our personal life's vision. When we're blocked in the sixth chakra, we deny what we see. We deny our imagination and have trouble believing that things could be different from how we perceive them to be. Although Ajna is about seeing things as they are, it's also about imagining how we can make things better. A blockage can keep us from opening to the possibility that we can manifest the change that we are capable if imagining. An excessively open sixth chakra can lead to delusion. When we are deluded, we see fantasy as reality; we lose the ability to discern the difference between what we observe and what we imagine. The archetype of this chakra is the Seer or Visionary. This is the part of ourselves that's able to see at all levels. Here we can let our powers of observation and intuition guide us to what is true. The negative sixth-chakra archetype is the Intellectual. The Intellectual may deny his or her natural intuition and see things only within a narrow set of socially dictated guidelines. The demon of Ajna is illusion. The affirmation of the sixth chakra is, "I have the right and the ability to see clearly."

The seventh chakra, whose Sanskrit name, Sahasrara, means "thousand-petaled lotus," is seen by some as being located at the crown of the head and by others as hovering just above it. This chakra is about consciousness. It's through Sahasrara that we see the oneness of things and our place in the cosmos. It's here at the seventh chakra that the consciousness within ourselves unites with the consciousness that we've seen as outside ourselves—the cosmic consciousness. Here we become one with all. Sahasrara literally means "the seat of the soul" and the seventh chakra is seen as the place that spirit first enters the body. When this chakra is closed, we become very limited in our ability to believe or have faith. Extreme spiritual skepticism can accompany a closed seventh chakra. At the same time, we may feel the need to be a know-it-all, to always be right. An excessively open Sahasrara may lead to spiritual addiction. We may have a need to believe in anything and everything, which can lead to becoming overwhelmed and confused. The archetype of the seventh chakra is the Sage or Guru. In Sanskrit the word *guru* means "one who leads us from dark to light." Sahasrara is where the guru within us abides, where our own wisdom, which can lead us from our delusion of separation to the truth of unity, awaits us. The negative archetype of the seventh chakra is the Egotist. This is the part of ourselves that feels it must hold on to the idea that we're separate—separate from others, from nature, and from our true selves. The demon of Sahasrara is attachment, the attachment to our separateness. The affirmation of the seventh chakra is, "I have the right to know or understand."

So why might it be important to be aware of these aspects of our chakras? In the tantric tradition, as well as in many of the traditions of energy healing, it's felt that the blocked energy or excessively open condition of a particular chakra relates to the negative physical, emotional, and spiritual aspects of that chakra, while the healthy, open flow of energy relates to its positive aspects. Whether the energy blockage preceded the manifestation of the negative aspects around a chakra, or the negative aspects lead to the blocked or excessive energy becomes a question only if we look at it in a Western, dualistic way. From a Taoist point of view, these things are inseparable; what causes one, causes the other and what heals one, heals the other. When we look at our feelings or behavior and recognize those parts of ourselves that feel negative to us, that are causing us suffering, we can use the chakra system to help us focus our healing intention. It's important to understand that we all hold within ourselves both the negative and positive archetypes and behavior patterns. We don't need to deny any of these parts of ourselves, but at the same time we want to reduce the suffering that some parts of ourselves bring to us. By not trying to push away the negative parts of ourselves, yet taking care to water the positive parts, we can watch as that which is causing us suffering quietly fades.

Here are a few sample ways to bring attention and healing to the chakras:

1. By concentrating on the location of the chakra
2. By keeping attention on the location while adding visualization of
   - the shape associated with the chakra
   - the color associated with the chakra
3. By chanting the bija or seed mantras associated with a particular chakra (see the Chakra Attributes table)
4. By repeating the affirmation of each chakra

Details about the attributes of each chakra can be found in the Chakra Attributes table on the next page. This table represents just one way to see and understand the chakra system. There are many others that I'm sure are equally valid.

CHAKRA ATTRIBUTES

Chakra	1st	2nd	3rd	4th	5th	6th	7th
Sanskrit name	Muladhara	Svadhis-thana	Manipura	Anahata	Vishuddha	Ajna	Sahasvava
Location	Base of spine	Sacrum, genitals	Solar plexus	Heart	Throat	Center of forehead	Crown of head
Meridians most affected	Kidney, Urinary Bladder	Kidney, Urinary Bladder	Stomach, Spleen	Heart, Small Intestine	Lung, Large Intestine	Conception, Governing	None recognized
Positive archetype	Earth mother	Lover	Hero	Healer	Artist, communicator	Seer	Sage, guru
Negative archetype	Victim	Martyr	Slave	Actor	Silent child	Excessive intellectual	Egotist
Demons	Fear	Guilt	Shame	Grief	Lies	Illusion	Attachment
Issues	Sense of belonging, security, survival, grounding	Sexuality, Pleasure / pain	Power, autonomy, self-esteem, confidence, will	Love, relationship, balance, compassion	Communication, speaking ones truth, self expression	Clarity, vision, imagination, seeing things as they really are	Growth, spirituality, eternity, mystery, relationship with the divine
Element	Earth	Water	Fire	Air	Ether	Light	None, pure consciousness
Color*	Red	Orange	Yellow	Green	Blue	Violet	Clear light
Shape	4-petaled lotus	6-petaled lotus	10-petaled lotus	12-petaled lotus	16-petaled lotus containing a triangle and circle	2-petaled lotus	1000-petaled lotus
Sound	Lam	Vam	Ram	Yam	Ham	Om	None
Affirmation	Right to be	Right to feel	Right to act	Right to love and be loved	Right to speak and be heard	Right to see clearly	Right to know, understand

---

*The colors that people see or sense for each chakra may vary depending on the level at which they are perceived—physical, astral, or causal. I have included the colors that are most commonly associated with each chakra.

YIN POSTURES, MERIDIANS, AND ENERGY CENTERS

People often wonder whether the chakras are the same as or different from the Chinese energy centers known as the *dan tian* (literally "elixir field"). According to Roger Jahnke, O.M.D., yoga is Indian qigong, and qigong is Chinese yoga, so the two systems are very similar, distinguished only by subtle differences of language and understanding. Like the Indian chakras, the three Chinese dan tian are centers where healing energy concentrates. The three dan tian are identical to three of the chakras.

The lower dan tian—associated with Earth Qi, the kidneys, and the metabolic organs—corresponds to the third, or umbilical, chakra. It produces, stores, and circulates the elixir for the body.

The middle dan tian—associated with Heart Mind Qi—corresponds to the fourth, or heart, chakra. It produces, stores, and circulates the elixir for the emotions and personality.

The upper dan tian—associated with Heaven Qi, the brain, and the glands in the brain—corresponds to the sixth, or third eye, chakra. It produces, stores, and circulates the elixir that radiates from the spirit.

To sum up the relationship of Yin Yoga postures to the stimulation of qi or prana in the Chinese and Indian energy systems, the following table lists which meridians, chakras, and dan tians are most often affected by which postures. These, of course, are generalizations but may be of interest to you in your pratice.

MERIDIANS AND ENERGY CENTERS AFFECTED BY EACH YIN POSTURE

Yin Postures	Meridians Affected	Energy Centers Affected
Half Butterfly	Urinary Bladder, Kidney, Liver, Gall Bladder	1st and 2nd Chakras
Shoelace	Kidney, Liver, Gall Bladder	1st and 2nd Chakras
Frog	Kidney, Urinary Bladder, Liver, Spleen	1st, 2nd, and 3rd Chakras, Lower Dan Tian
Seal	Kidney, Urinary Bladder, Stomach, Spleen	1st and 3rd Chakras, Lower Dan Tian
Butterfly	Kidney, Liver	1st and 2nd Chakras
Forward Bend	Urinary Bladder	1st Chakra
Dragonfly	Kidney, Urinary Bladder, Liver	1st and 2nd Chakras
Square Pose	Urinary Bladder, Gall Bladder	1st and 2nd Chakras
Swan	Kidney, Urinary Bladder, Stomach, Spleen, Gall Bladder	1st, 2nd, and 3rd Chakras, Lower Dan Tian
Sleeping Swan	Stomach, Spleen, Gall Bladder	3rd Chakra, Lower Dan Tian
Saddle	Stomach, Spleen, Urinary Bladder, Kidney	1st, 2nd, and 3rd Chakras, Lower Dan Tian
Spinal Twist	Gall Bladder	1st, 2nd, and 4th Chakras, Middle Dan Tian

Part 2

Practicing Yin Yoga

GUIDELINES FOR A YIN YOGA PRACTICE

There are two guidelines I use when practicing Yin Yoga:

1. **Assume the suggested or chosen posture and allow yourself to move into the pose to a bearable but challenging edge.** You will probably feel some intensity of sensation and that's fine as long as it feels safe to you and your breathing remains free and smooth. Ultimately, it is most important to be able to be at ease in the posture. Let your muscles relax without striving to go deeper into the pose, accepting where you are in your body at that moment.
2. **Allowing your muscles to relax and feeling them melt around your bones, remain still and hold the pose for the determined time.** For most people five minutes works well. If you fall deeper into the posture as you hold it, that's fine, but it's important to be sure that you're not striving to go deeper into the pose. Let any layers of holding drop away as you relax. Keep checking in with your breath; if you notice

that you're not able to breathe comfortably, you may be trying too hard. Just back off a little until you can breathe in a relaxed way while still maintaining a feeling of some intensity in the areas that the pose targets for you. In Yin Yoga, as in any physical activity, it's important to listen to your body and honor its wisdom—if ever a pose feels injurious be sure to back off or come out of the pose. Only you can know for certain the type of practice that is best for your body.

In this book and card set I've included fourteen postures. This doesn't mean that these are the only yoga poses that can be part of a Yin practice. Any posture that you feel you can hold safely for an extended time, while keeping your mind focused and your muscles relaxed, can be done as a Yin posture.

THE YIN YOGA POSTURES

The fourteen postures in *The Yin Yoga Kit* are all done on the floor so that the muscles can relax and allow the deep connective tissue surrounding the lower back, the pelvis, and the joints of the femurs to be gently stretched. This stretching helps to maintain the health of the connective tissue and encourages the free flow of qi through the six meridians that pass through the hips. By promoting the flow of energy through the meridians, Yin Yoga helps us to maintain our physical health, as well as our emotional and energetic balance. For each posture that follows, I have included some of the emotional and energetic attributes that are associated with the meridians stimulated by that pose. The attributes listed are not meant to be an all-inclusive guide to the meridians; they are just a suggestion of some of the ways the posture may affect you by encouraging energy flow in those meridians. You will find more detail on the meridians and their effects in the meridian chapter beginning on page 13.

I have noted the chakras affected by each pose as well. Most of the Yin Yoga postures help to energize some combination of the first three chakras: Muladhara, located at the base of the spine, Svadisthana, located at the sacrum and genitals, and Manipura, located at the solar plexus. When the first three chakras are healthy, we can more easily feel grounded and secure, be more comfortable with our sexuality, have more capacity to feel pleasure and pain, and can reclaim our confidence and self-esteem.

Above all, Yin Yoga is a gentle practice that teaches us to relax and accept ourselves just as we are. Some of these poses may feel challenging to you, especially at the beginning of your practice. I have included descriptions and photographs of variations and adaptations for each pose (including the use of props) that can help you get comfortable in the postures, even if your flexibility is quite limited.

Feel free to do the postures, in any order that feels good to you. Many people like to alternate forward bends and back bends as they practice, others choose poses to stimulate specific meridians. You might feel tired one day and energized another, which will affect the poses you choose to do. Experiment and see what feels best for you on any given day.

The fourteen postures in order of appearance are as follows:

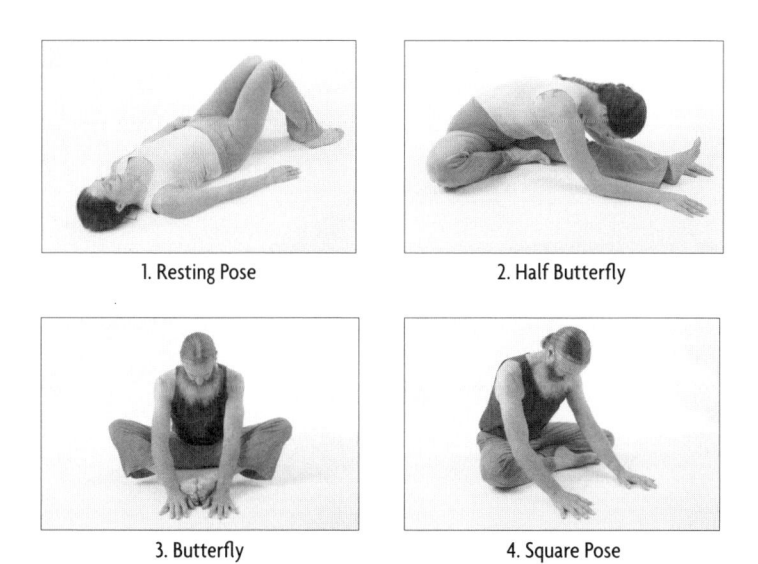

1. Resting Pose

2. Half Butterfly

3. Butterfly

4. Square Pose

5. Shoelace

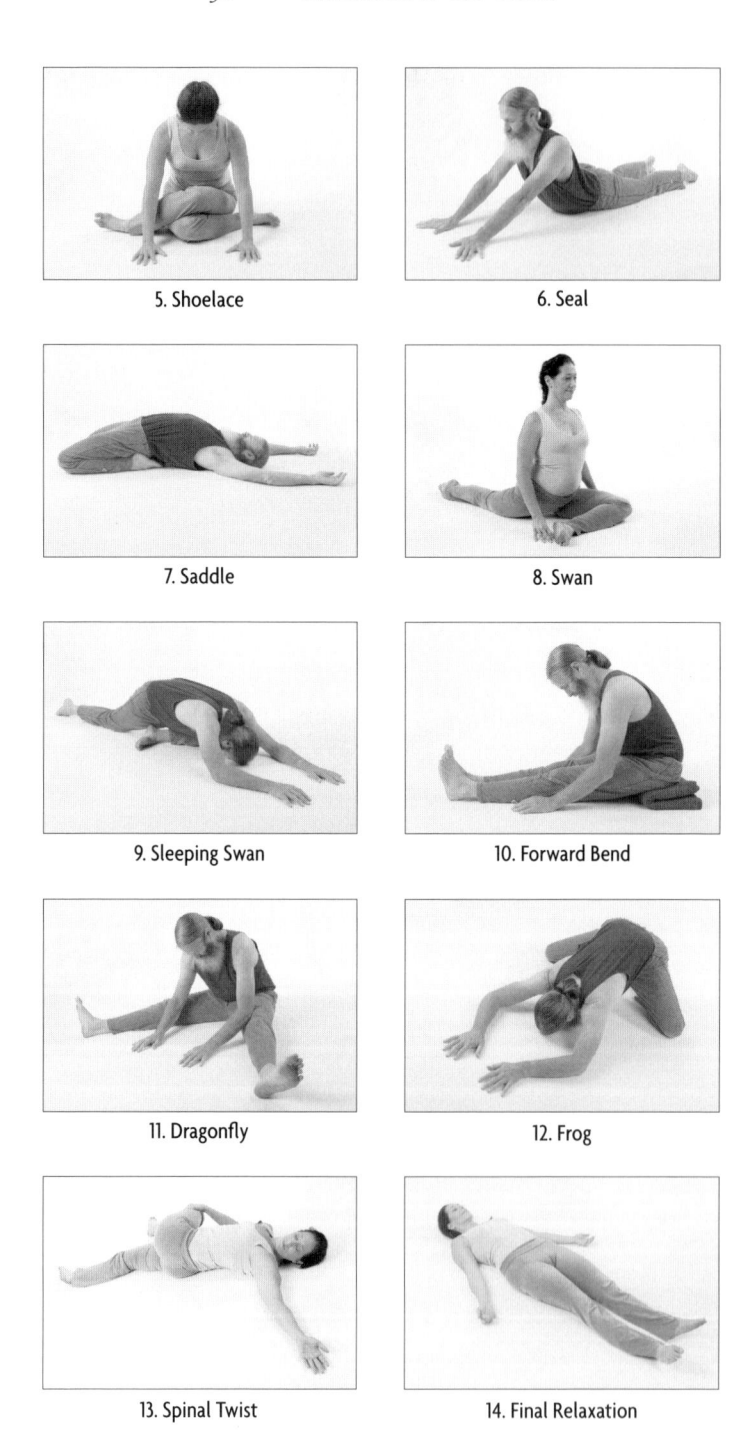

6. Seal

7. Saddle

8. Swan

9. Sleeping Swan

10. Forward Bend

11. Dragonfly

12. Frog

13. Spinal Twist

14. Final Relaxation

Resting Pose

Lying on your back, bend your knees up to a right angle, keeping your feet flat on the floor, hip-width apart. Relax the muscles around your lower back and hips and let your knees fall toward one another. Direct your breath to any place you feel holding, particularly the muscles that affect the movement of the lower spine, the pelvis, and the femurs. Let your arms relax wherever they feel most comfortable.

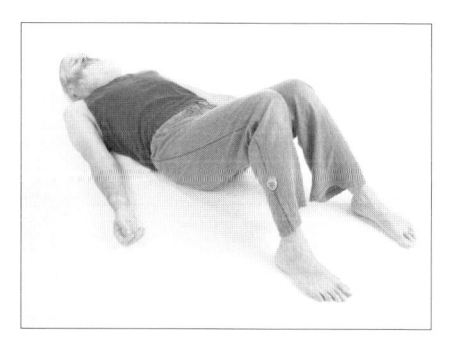

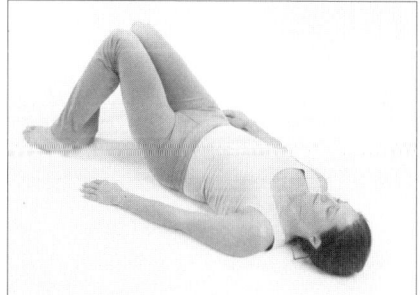

Variations

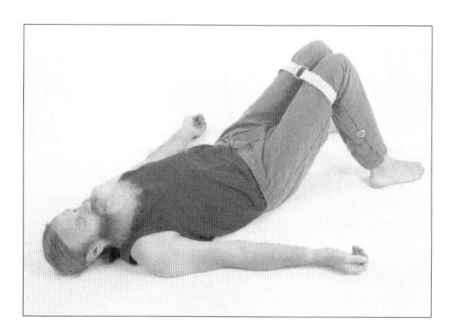

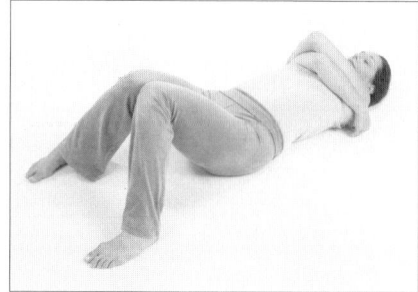

Try varying the position of your feet, bringing them closer to your hips or moving them farther away, to allow your femurs to relax into your hip sockets. Adjust the width of your feet to allow your knees to rest against each other without effort. You can use a strap to hold your knees together if they tend to fall open. For some people, a cushion between the knees helps the hips to relax. Play around with the position of your arms to allow your shoulders to soften. You may want to cross your arms over your chest, visualizing them as empty shirtsleeves.

Benefits

Resting Pose helps relax the iliopsoas muscle—the muscle connecting the lower spine, pelvis, and femurs—which is a place where we often hold tension. Because of our hectic lifestyles and the high level of stress in modern life, it is very important to take the time to bring attention to this area, letting our body know that we are safe and it's all right to relax. By allowing the femurs to gently fall back into their sockets, we allow all the muscles in the hips to relax. This is a good pose with which to begin a Yin Yoga practice.

Meridians Stimulated

By relaxing and bringing our attention and breath to the pelvic area, we can stimulate all six meridians that pass through this area—Stomach, Gall Bladder, Kidney, Liver, Spleen, and Urinary Bladder. Encouraging the free flow of energy to these major organs can help them to properly do their job in physically supporting the body. When energy flows smoothly to these organs they will remain in harmony. When the organs are in harmony we can most easily embrace their positive emotional attributes, such as compassion, decisiveness, courage, wisdom, kindness, and creativity. (See the table on page 18 for more details on the organ meridians and their attributes.)

The Yin Yoga Postures • 39

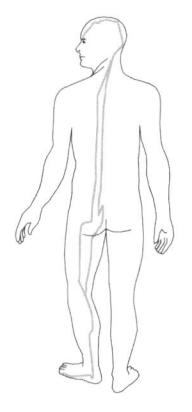

Urinary Bladder meridian

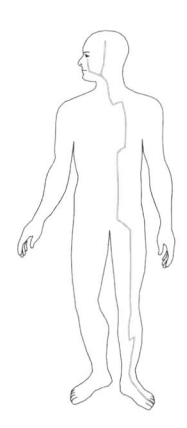

Stomach meridian

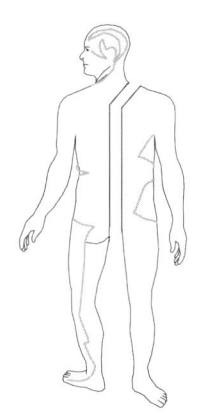

Gall Bladder meridian

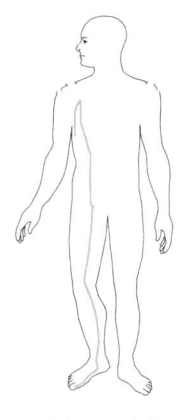

Spleen meridian

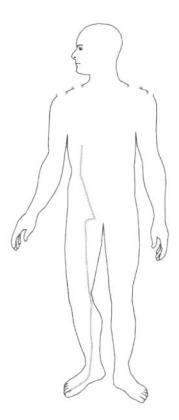

Liver meridian

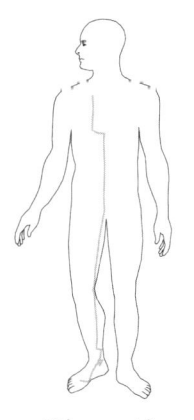

Kidney meridian

Chakras Affected

Whichever you choose to focus on

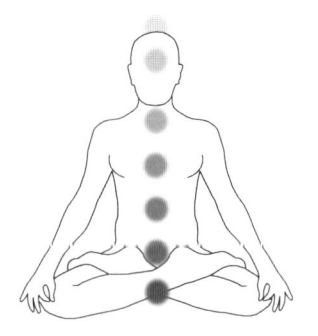

Cautions

None

Half Butterfly

Sitting with your legs extended, bend one leg, bringing the sole of that foot to rest on the opposite inner thigh. Beginning with a straight back, lean forward as far as you can without pushing, then, with an attitude of relaxed acceptance, let your back round. Repeat on the other side.

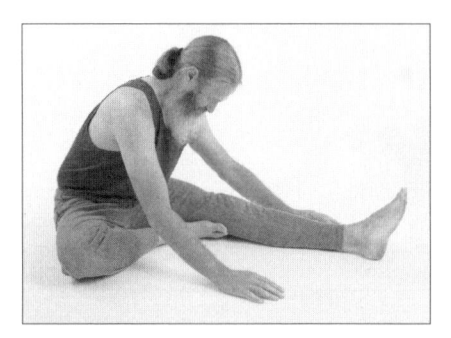

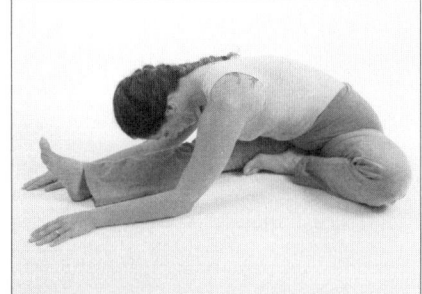

Variations

Half Butterfly can be a stretch for the whole back if you stretch straight forward or a gentle side stretch when you stretch toward the extended leg. Most people find it useful to use a cushion under their sitz bones* to maintain a healthy pelvic tilt. Use a cushion under your bent knee to relieve hip stress. Bend the straight leg slightly to release your hamstrings in order to allow a deeper forward bend. This will also help relieve discomfort in the back of that knee and relieve stress to the sciatic nerve.

---

*I use the phrase *sitz bones* throughout *The Yin Yoga Kit* to refer to what are anatomically called the ischial tuberosities. These are not really bones, in themselves, but are the portion of the ishium, or pelvis, that is designed to provide a stable platform when we sit. You can locate the sitz bones by reaching under your buttocks as you sit in a chair. Near or at the point where you contact your chair you will feel them as two bony protrusions. It's important in any sitting posture to be sure that you are firmly planted on these two bones, not slouched back or tipped forward. Proper alignment will allow you to sit stably and comfortably and to feel a strong, grounded connection to the earth.

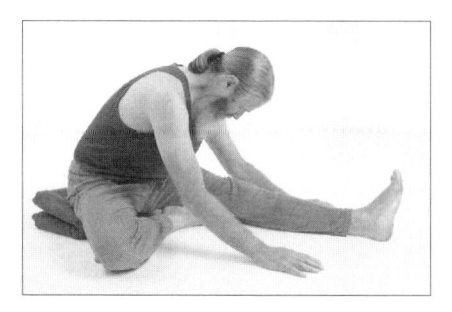

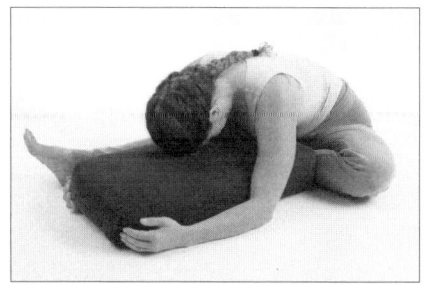

Place blocks on either side of the straightened knee, with bolsters or cushions on top on which to rest your arms, chest, or head without putting uncomfortable weight on the knee.

Benefits

Half Butterfly is a stretch for the whole back. It also stretches the groin and hip on the bent-leg side and the hamstrings on the straight leg.

Meridians Stimulated

Half Butterfly stimulates the, Liver, Kidney, Gall Bladder, and Urinary Bladder meridians. The Liver meridian is considered to be the seat of human kindness, so stimulating it helps us to find kindness in ourselves. Stimulation of the Kidney meridian calms fear, while bringing energy to the Gall Bladder meridian helps us to have courage. Because energy blockages in the Urinary Bladder meridian usually manifest physically, stimulating it will help prevent urinary problems, such as difficulty urinating, incontinence, or uncomfortable or burning urination. A harmonious Urinary Bladder meridian also supports the positive emotional attributes of the Kidney meridian.

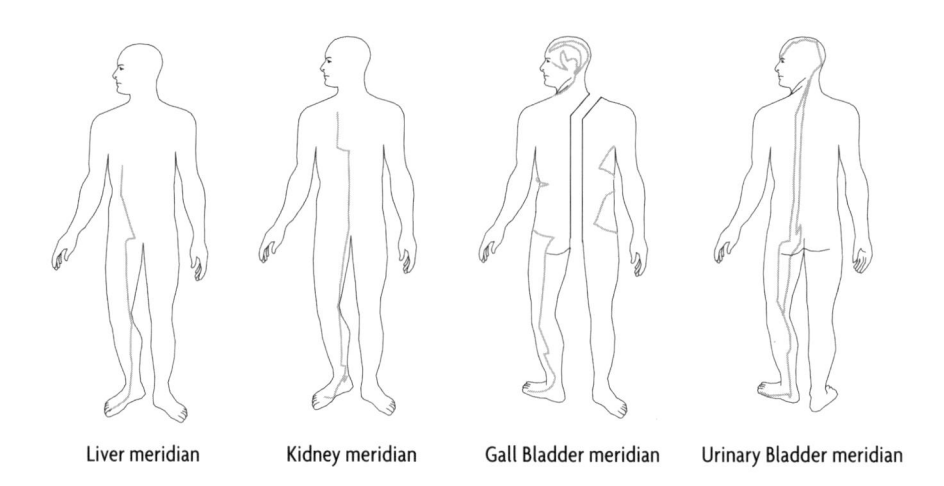

Liver meridian   Kidney meridian   Gall Bladder meridian   Urinary Bladder meridian

Chakras Affected
First (Muladhara) and Second (Svadhisthana)

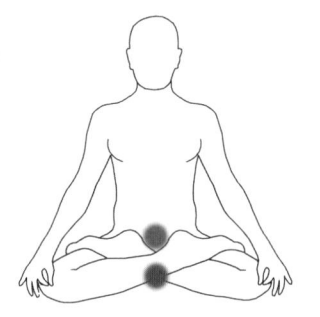

Cautions
Maintain a pelvic tilt in Half Butterfly by using cushions and/or bending the extended knee.

Butterfly

Sit on your sitz bones with the soles of your feet together about a foot from your body. Either remain upright or, if the flexibility of your hips allows it, lean forward with a straight back to your comfortable edge, and then let your back gently round.

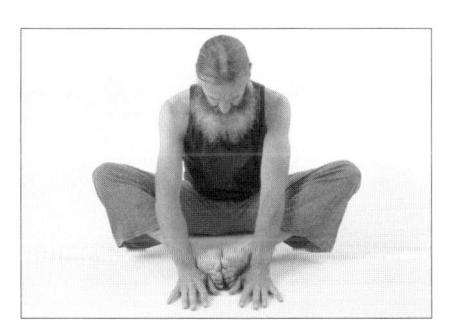

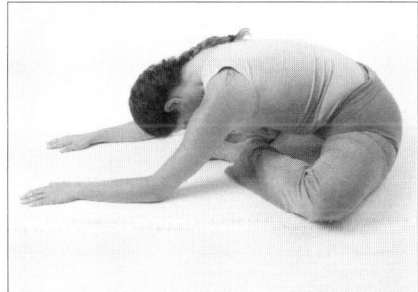

Variations

Many people will need a cushion under their sitz bones to keep their sacrum from tilting back. Use cushions under your knees to relieve hip stress. Use cushions on the floor in front of you in order to rest your head and ease any strain to your neck. Try moving your heels toward or away from your torso and feel how it changes the stretch.

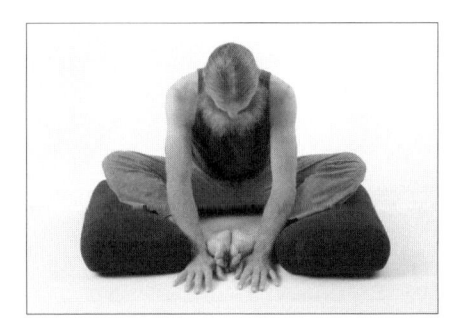

Benefits

Butterfly is a good stretch for the back and groin. It also opens the hips.

Meridians Stimulated

Butterfly stimulates the Liver and Kidney meridians. Harmonious Liver meridian energy allows anger to transform into kindness. The kidney is home of jing, our essence and potential. Experiencing our true essence can bring us to a place of kindness and replace fear with wisdom.

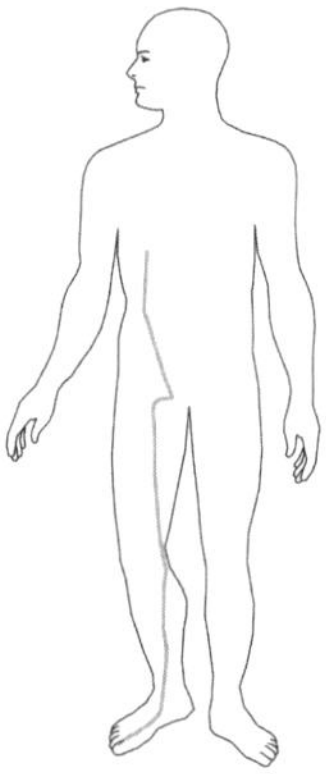

Liver meridian 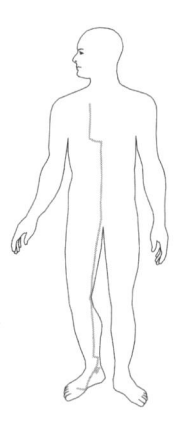   Kidney meridian

Chakras Affected

First (Muladhara) and Second (Svadhisthana)

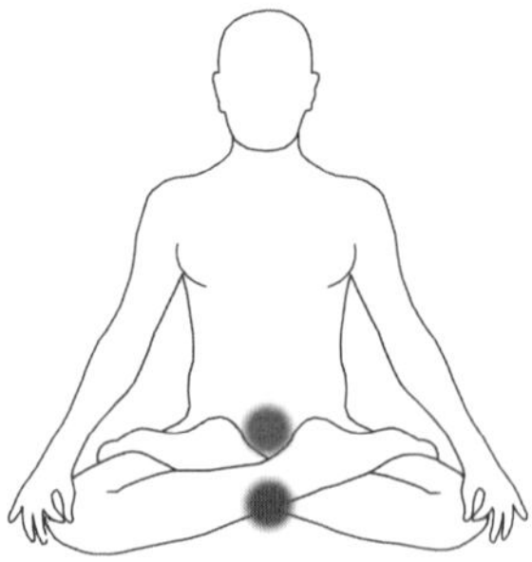

Cautions

Be aware of any strain to your neck in Butterfly. Be sure to maintain a sacral/pelvic tilt.

Square Pose

Sitting cross-legged, place one ankle either on the opposite thigh or in front of the opposite shin. With a straight back, lean forward to your comfortable edge; then let your back gently round.

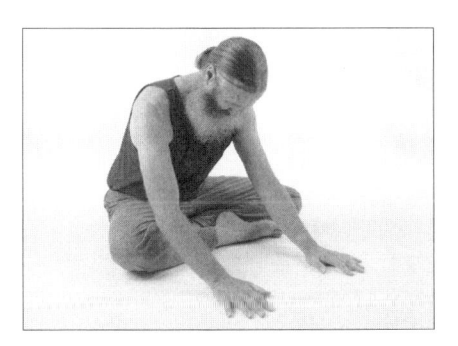

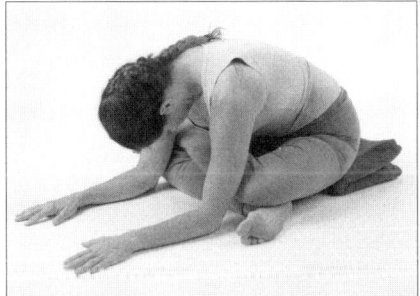

Variations

Use a cushion under your sitz bones to increase your forward pelvic tilt. It's fine to use cushions under your knees to take the stress off your hips, allowing the muscles to relax. You may also rest your head or forearms on a cushion to ease neck or shoulder strain.

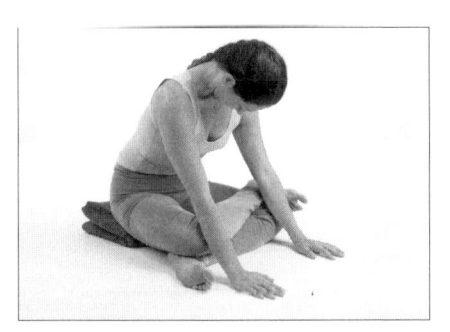

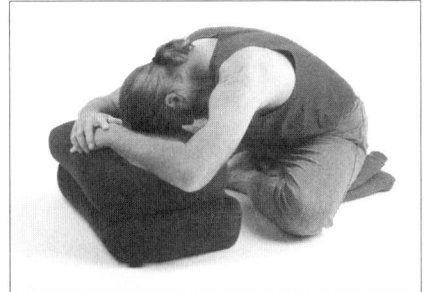

Benefits

Square Pose stretches the hips and groin as well as the whole back.

Meridians Stimulated

Square Pose stimulates the Gall Bladder and Urinary Bladder meridians. The gall bladder controls courage and decisiveness. Feelings of hesitancy and disregard for caution are signs of disharmony in this meridian. A harmonious flow of Gall Bladder meridian energy can transform these feelings into their opposites. Because a branch of the Urinary Bladder meridian enters the kidney, stimulation of this meridian will affect the health of the kidney as well and promote its positive emotional attributes, encouraging kindness and calming fear.

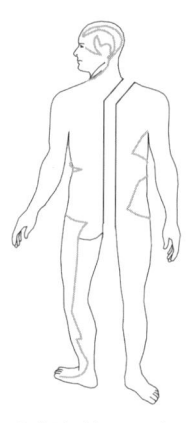

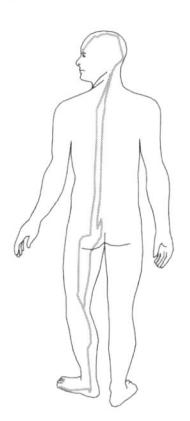

Gall Bladder meridian   Urinary Bladder meridian

Chakras Affected

First (Muladhara) and Second (Svadhisthana)

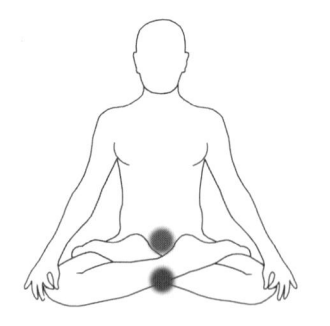

Cautions

Maintain a forward pelvic tilt. Be aware of any excessive stress to the knees in Square Pose.

Shoelace

The easiest way to get into shoelace is to start on all fours. From there, slide one knee behind the other—your right foot will now be to your left and your left foot to your right. Now sit back so that you're sitting between your ankles—your knees will be stacked one on top of the other. If you comfortably can, lean forward. Repeat with the other leg on top.

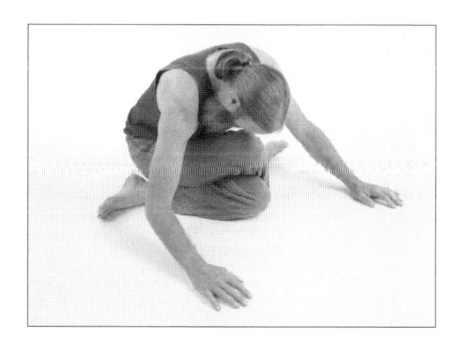

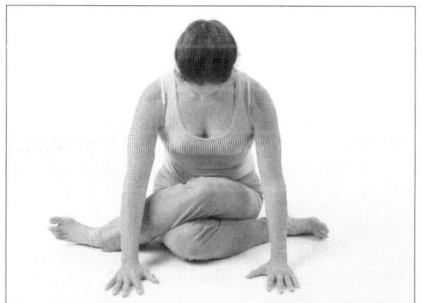

Variations

Use a cushion under your sitz bones to help level your torso and establish a healthy pelvic/sacral tilt. This is especially important for those who remain nearly vertical in this pose. Square Pose may be substituted for those who find Shoelace too intense. You may do this pose with a straight lower leg if your knee feels overstressed.

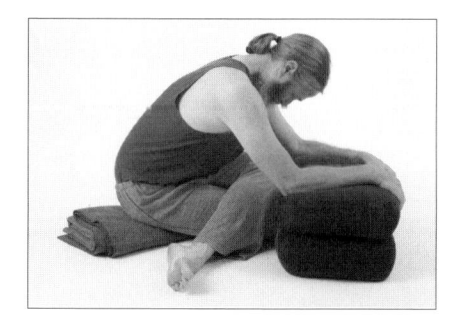

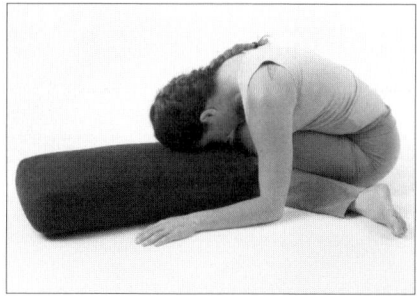

Benefits
Shoelace brings opening to the lower back (lumbar spine) and hips.

Meridians Stimulated
Shoelace stimulates the Kidney, Liver, and Gall Bladder meridians. Increasing the flow of qi to the Kidney meridian puts us in touch with our true essence, encouraging gentleness and calming fear. Stimulating the Liver meridian encourages the flow of qi throughout the whole body and encourages kindness. When our Gall Bladder meridian is in harmony, we can more easily be courageous and decisive.

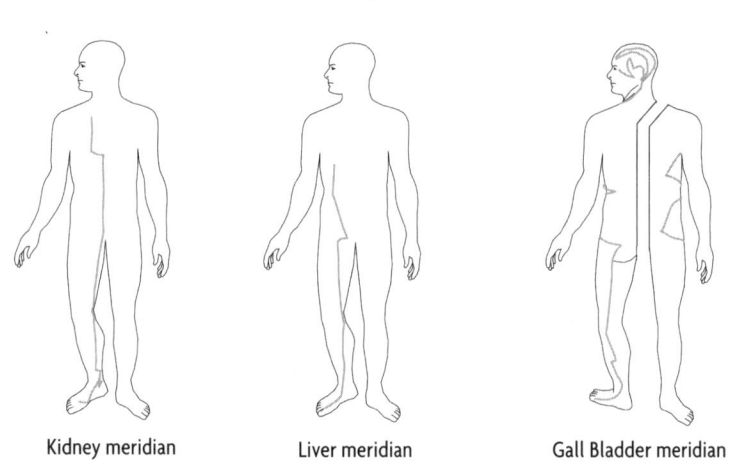

Kidney meridian   Liver meridian   Gall Bladder meridian

Chakras Affected
First (Muladhara) and Second (Svadhisthana)

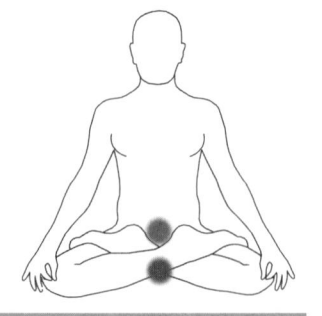

Cautions
Be sure to maintain some forward tilt to the sacrum in Shoelace.

Seal

Lying on your belly with arms extended, raise your torso to your comfortable edge, hands turned out at approximately 30 degrees (thumbs should be more or less parallel). Relax your shoulders and let your belly droop toward the floor, visualizing your spine as a string of pearls hanging gracefully from the back of your head to your tailbone. If it feels comfortable and safe for you, try to relax your buttocks.

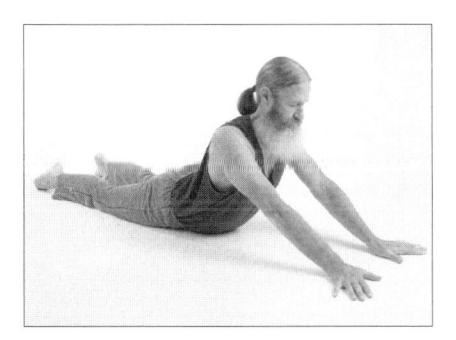

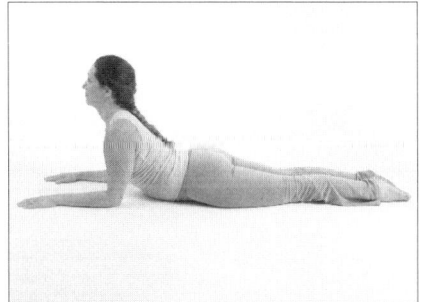

Variations

To ease the intensity to the lower back, adjust the angle of your arms or lower yourself to your forearms, resting them on the floor or on a cushion or bolster. This will lower your torso, giving you a gentler back bend and allowing you to more easily relax your shoulders and arms. Spreading your feet wide apart or bringing your legs closer together will change the way you experience this pose. Neither way is inherently better; they're just different. Experiment. (After all, they are your legs.)

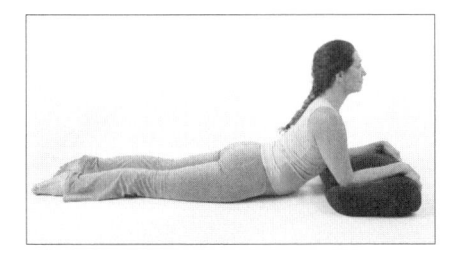

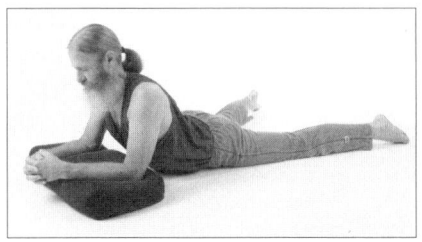

Benefits

Seal helps to reestablish the natural curve of the lumbar spine and may help relieve lower-back pain and stiffness.

Meridians Stimulated

Seal stimulates the Stomach, Spleen, Kidney, and Urinary Bladder meridians. The stomach is the home of sympathy and compassion, so a harmonious Stomach meridian encourages these emotions. When the stomach Meridian is blocked or restricted, we may begin to feel a nervousness that can become moodiness, suspicion, paranoia, or even the source of violent and explosive behavior. We can also begin to lose confidence, letting ourselves be too easily influenced by others. The spleen is where we hold the awareness of our own potentials. A harmonious Spleen meridian helps us see the options in our lives, helps us weigh all our possibilities, and motivates us to realize our creative potential. Disharmonies in the Spleen meridian lead to excessive worry and indecision. Stimulating the Kidney meridian helps to put us in touch with our jing—our own true essence—encouraging wisdom and gentleness. A harmonious Urinary Bladder meridian supports the positive emotional attributes of the Kidney meridian, as well as promoting physical health for the bladder.

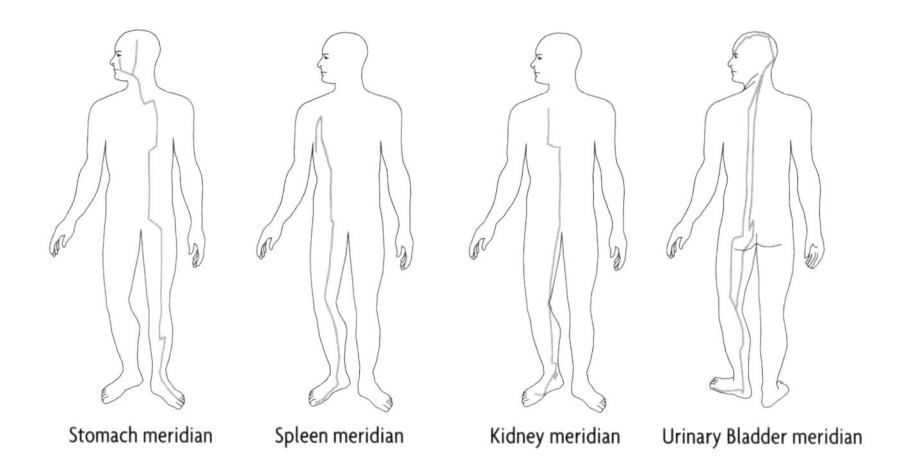

Stomach meridian — Spleen meridian — Kidney meridian — Urinary Bladder meridian

Chakras Affected

First (Muladhara) and Third (Manipura)

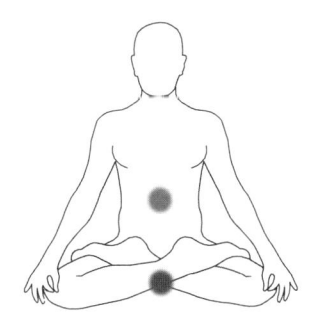

Cautions

If you allow your neck to relax, be sure the weight of your head doesn't cause neck strain.

Saddle

Kneeling with your hips between your heels, lean back to your comfortable edge using your arms, cushions, or the floor for support. When you're not using your arms for support, you can keep them at your sides or extend them over your head.

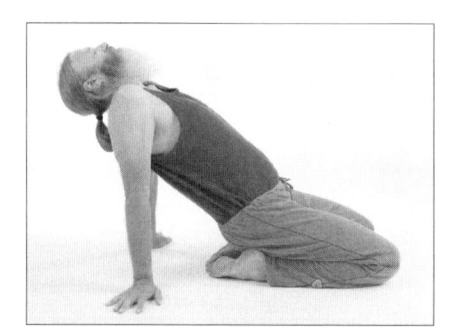

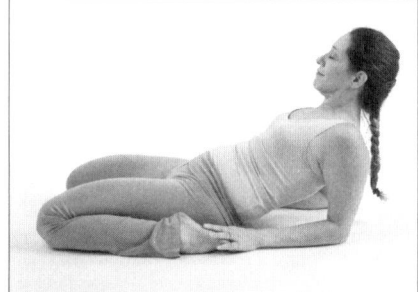

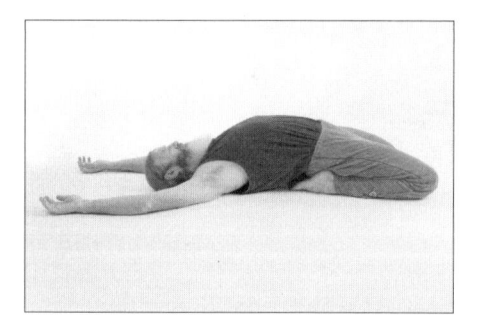

Variations

It is very common for people to use props in Saddle. If going all the way to the floor creates too much stress on your ankles, knees, lower back, or sacral area, you can stack cushions or bolsters to support yourself. Note that the bolsters shown in the illustrations are under the shoulders. If you place the support under your lower back, the posture becomes more of a restorative pose. Although it can be very beneficial, it doesn't have as strong an effect on the lumbar spine or on the associated meridians.

Use as much support as you need. You can even lean back against a sofa or an armchair. A rolled-up towel or mat under the front of the ankles or behind your knees may relieve strain in these areas.

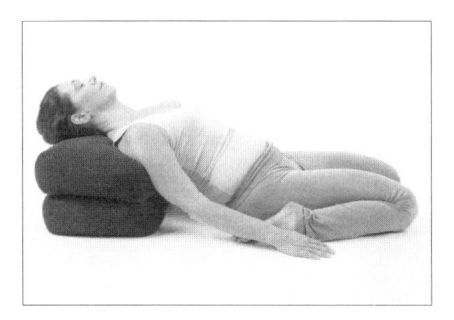

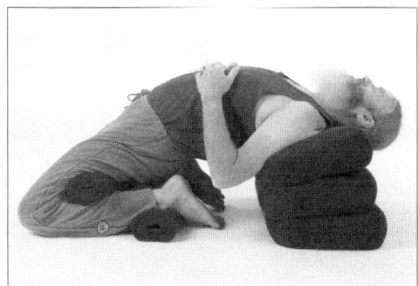

Benefits

Saddle reestablishes the lumbar curve and helps to bring the sacrum up and into its home in the ilium. This postural correction energizes the body and helps to counter the effects of aging and our sedentary lifestyles. For many people, Saddle helps ease lower-back pain.

Meridians Stimulated

Saddle stimulates the Stomach, Spleen, Urinary Bladder, and Kidney meridians. A free flow of qi to the Stomach meridian encourages sympathy and compassion, while a blocked Stomach meridian can lead to nervousness, moodiness, paranoia, or even violence. A harmonious Spleen meridian opens our creative potential by helping us see our options and weigh all of our possibilities, while a blocked flow of qi to the spleen contributes to worry and indecisiveness. A free flow of qi in the Kidney meridian encourages our inner wisdom and gentleness. A harmonious Urinary Bladder meridian promotes urinary tract health and lends additional support to the positive emotional attributes of the Kidney meridian.

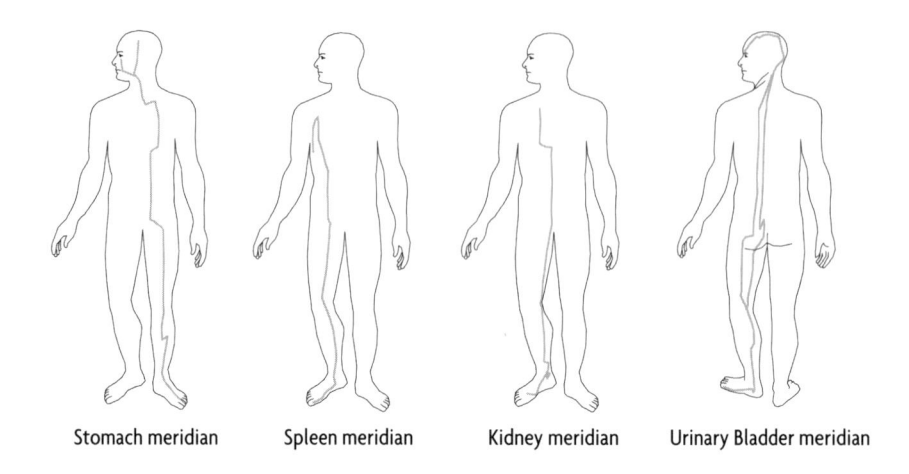

Stomach meridian   Spleen meridian   Kidney meridian   Urinary Bladder meridian

Chakras Affected
First (Muladhara), Second (Svadhisthana), and Third (Manipura)

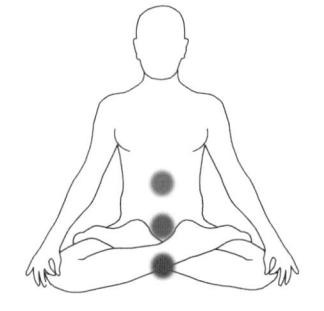

Cautions
Saddle is a powerful pose so be sure to honor your body's wisdom, particularly if you feel stress on the inside of the knees.

Swan

Start on all fours. Slide your left knee forward toward your left hand and your right knee back away from your right hand. Bring your left foot toward your right hand as far as is comfortable. Let your torso go into a gentle back bend, supported by your extended arms. Repeat on the other side.

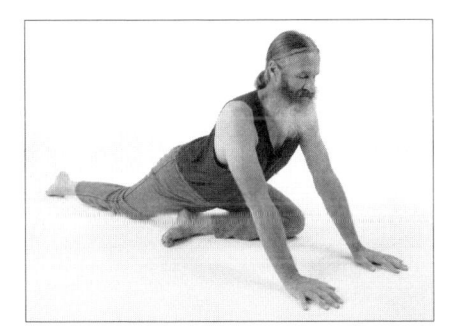

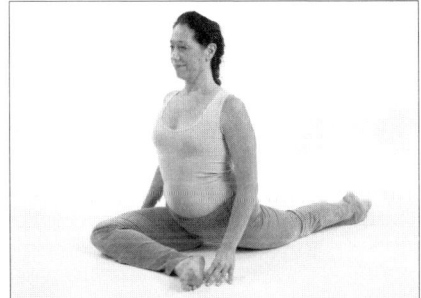

Variations

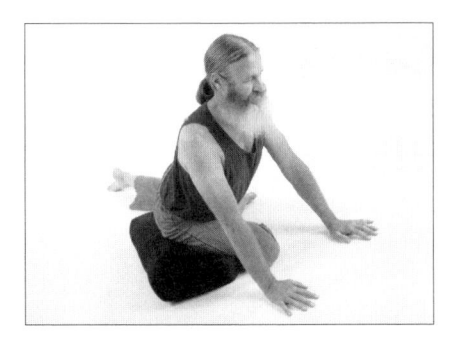

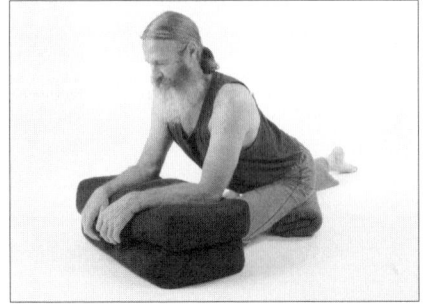

Use cushions or blankets for support under the hip of your bent leg as needed. If you feel too much stress on your wrists, arms, or shoulders you can use a bolster under your forearms. You can hold Swan for the entire timed period or partway through you can drape forward into Sleeping Swan. You may also deepen the pose by bending the knee of your straight leg to lift your foot off the floor. Then reach back on that side and grab your foot with your hand. For a deeper back bend and greater hip extension on your straight leg, extend both hands over your head.

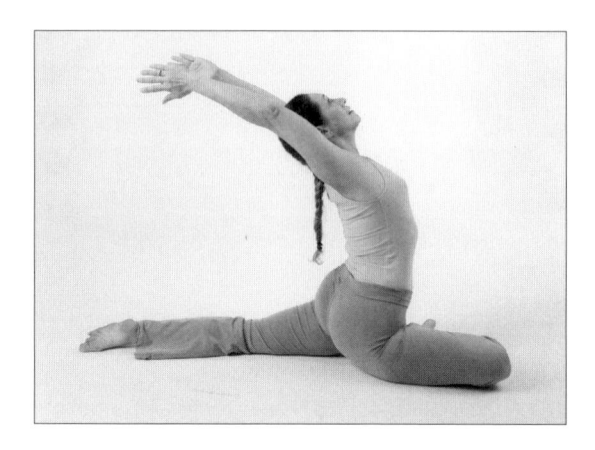

Benefits

Swan stretches the hip flexors, hip rotators, groin, and lumbar spine.

Meridians Stimulated

Swan stimulates the Gall Bladder, Stomach, Spleen, Kidney, and Urinary Bladder meridians, helping us feel our own courage, compassion, creativity, and wisdom. It also helps bring physical health to the urinary tract. This posture energizes and opens the mind and body.

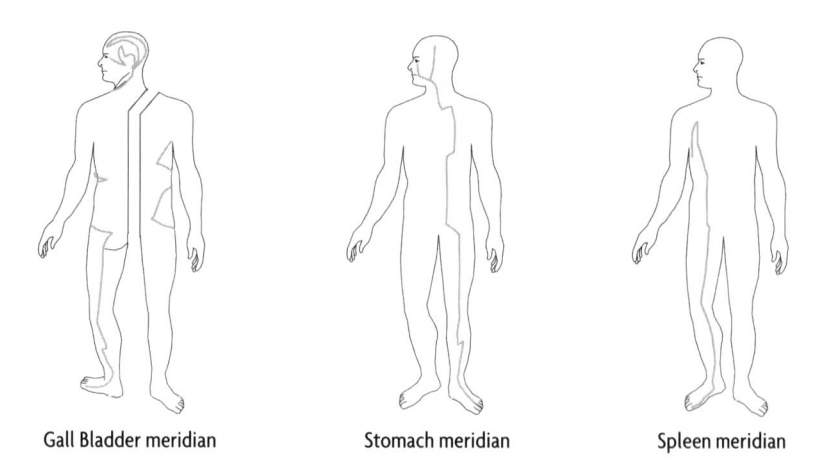

Gall Bladder meridian Stomach meridian Spleen meridian

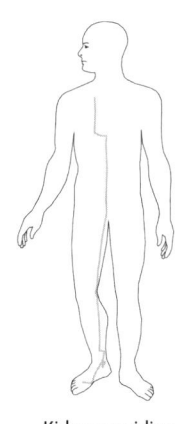

Kidney meridian 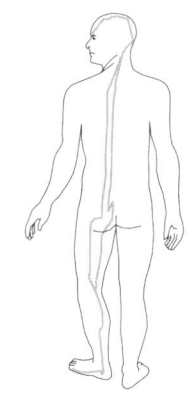   Urinary Bladder meridian

Chakras Affected
First (Muladhara), Second (Svadhisthana), and Third (Manipura)

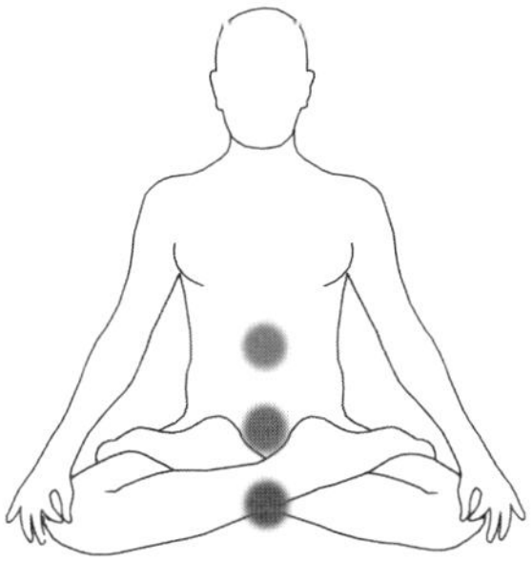

Cautions
Be aware of excess stress to the bent knee or the sacroiliac joint (lower back and tailbone area). Be gentle with your neck.

Sleeping Swan

Starting on all fours, slide your left knee forward toward your left hand and your right knee back away from your right hand. Bring your left foot toward your right hand as far as comfortable. Drape your torso forward, relaxing into the stretch. Repeat on the other side.

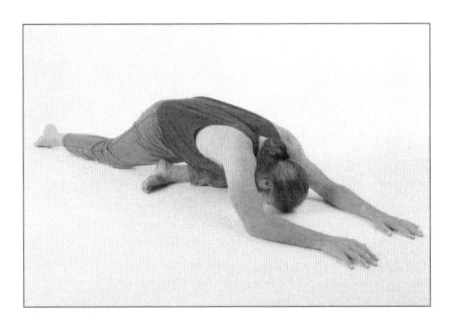

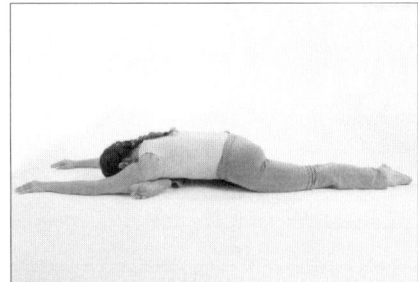

Variations

Use cushions anywhere you can think of to make the posture more comfortable. Try cushions or blankets under your chest or under the thigh of your bent leg. If you bend the straight leg you may find that it changes the stretch on that hip. Sleeping Swan is often done from Swan posture. You can combine Swan and Sleeping Swan as one posture by changing from one to the other partway through your timed period.

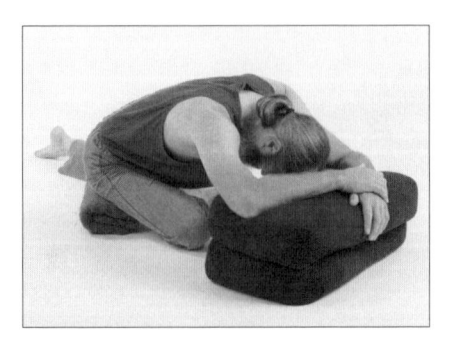

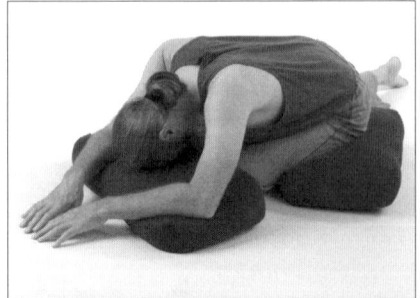

Benefits
Sleeping Swan stretches the hip flexors, hip rotators, and groin.

Meridians Stimulated
Sleeping Swan stimulates the Gall Bladder, Stomach, and Spleen meridians. A healthy flow of qi in the Gall Bladder meridian helps us to feel courageous and decisive. A harmonious Stomach meridian encourages sympathy and compassion, while a harmonious Spleen meridian opens us to our creative potential.

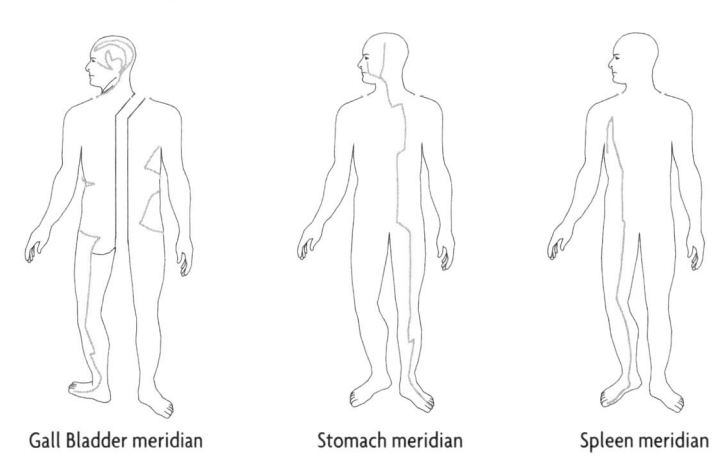

Gall Bladder meridian   Stomach meridian   Spleen meridian

Chakras Affected
Third (Manipura)

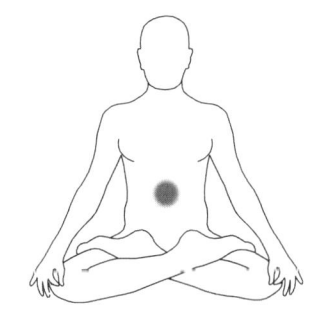

Cautions
Be aware of excess stress to the bent knee or the sacroiliac joint (lower back and tailbone area).

Forward Bend

Start in a seated position with your legs extended. Keeping your back straight, bend forward until you can't go any farther. Then let your back relax into a soft curve. Don't strive to go deeper. Just breathe and relax; enjoy being just where you are.

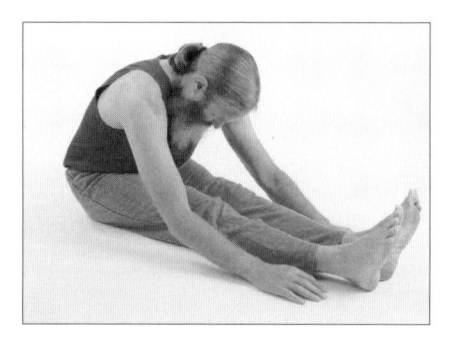

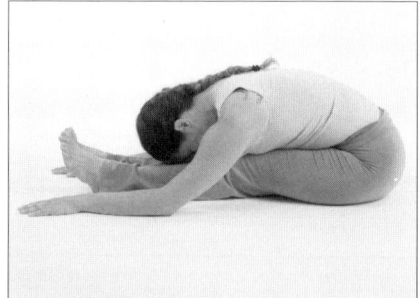

Variations

Many people benefit from using a cushion under their sitz bones to help keep a healthy sacral tilt. If your hamstrings are tight, it's fine to bend your knees, allowing you to use gravity to get deeper into the forward bend. If you're very deep in the posture and your neck feels compromised, you can use cushions to support your head.

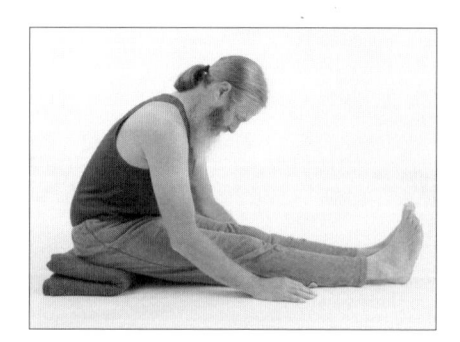

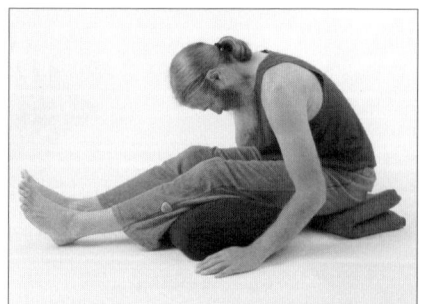

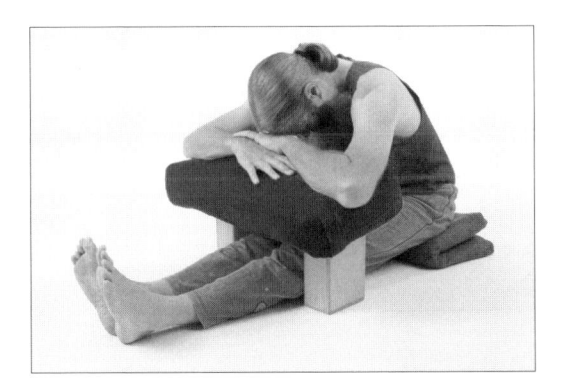

Benefits

Forward Bend stretches the whole back of the body and releases physical and mental tension. With the legs straight, it's also an effective hamstring stretch.

Meridians Stimulated

Forward Bend stimulates the Urinary Bladder meridian, encouraging the health of the whole urinary tract. Because a branch of the Urinary Bladder meridian enters the kidney, stimulation of this meridian will lend additional support the to the health of the kidney. Harmony in the kidney helps bring us home to our true essence.

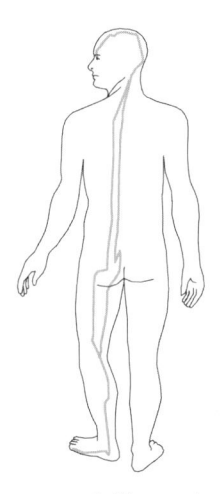

Urinary Bladder meridian

Chakras Affected
First (Muladhara) and Second (Svadhisthana)

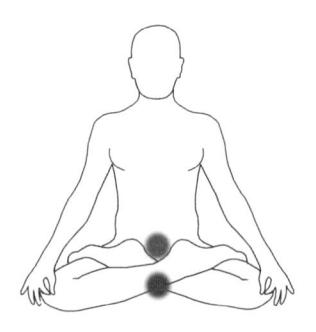

Cautions
Be sure that your pelvis is tilted forward at least slightly to prevent undo stress to your sacral area. All seated forward bends are potentially painful and injurious for people with sciatica.

Dragonfly

Start by sitting with your legs straight in front of you as though preparing for a seated Forward Bend. Then spread them as wide as is comfortable, coming into whatever sort of split works for you at the moment. Either stay as you are or, with a straight back, lean forward to your own edge. When you reach it, let your back round.

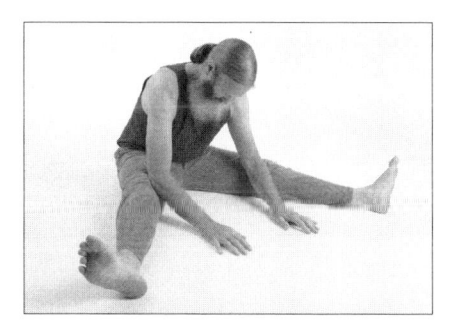

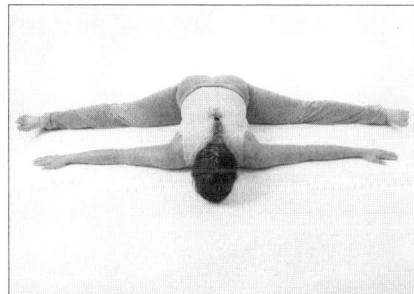

Variations

For many people, a cushion under the buttocks is necessary to maintain a forward tilt of the pelvis. The knees can be bent slightly to release the hamstrings and ease the stress to the inside of the knees. Try using a cushion under each knee if your knees need support. Rest your head or chin on cushions or on your hands to relieve the stress to your neck.

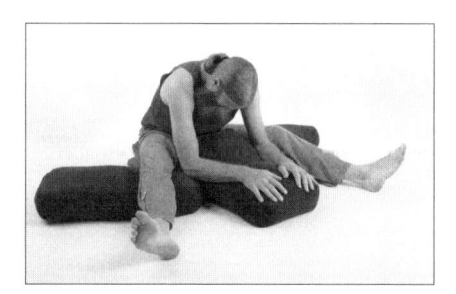

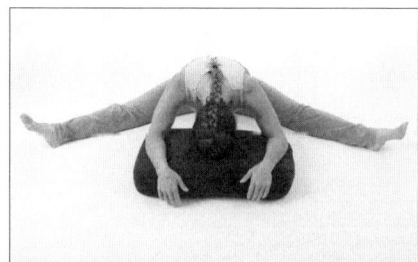

Benefits

Dragonfly stretches the lower back, hips, and hamstrings.

Meridians Stimulated

Dragonfly stimulates the Kidney, Liver, and Urinary Bladder meridians, putting us in touch with our true essence, encouraging wisdom and kindness, and helping to calm fear and anger.

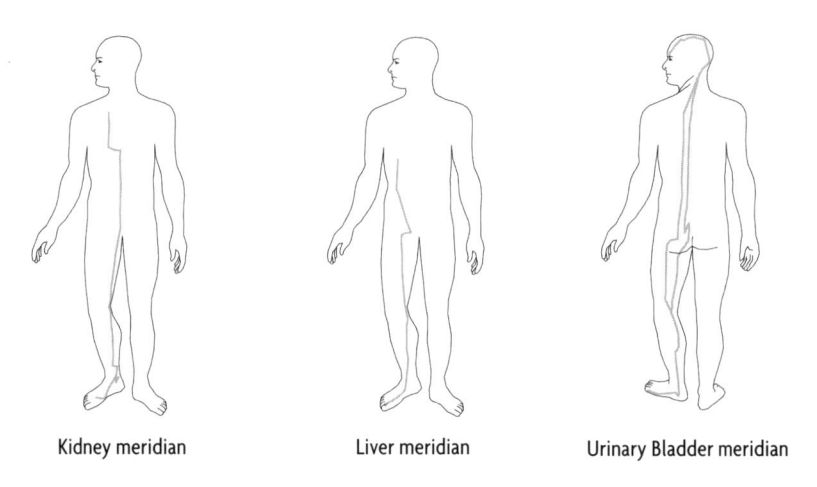

Kidney meridian   Liver meridian   Urinary Bladder meridian

Chakras Affected

First (Muladhara) and Second (Svadhisthana)

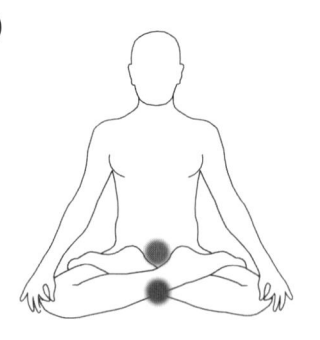

Cautions

Be sure to maintain some pelvic tilt. Dragonfly is a challenging forward bend. Relax and be compassionate with yourself.

Frog

Starting on all fours, spread your knees as wide as you comfortably can and sink back onto your heels in a wide-knee Child's Pose. You can keep your arms at your sides or stretch them over your head.

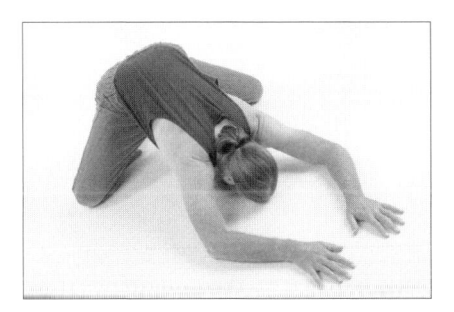

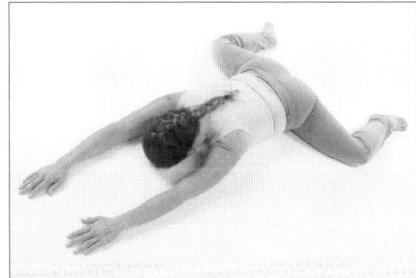

Variations

You can use bolsters under your forehead to support your neck, or under your chest, belly, or pelvis to reduce strain on your inner thighs. If you're very flexible, you may be able to sink straight to the floor.

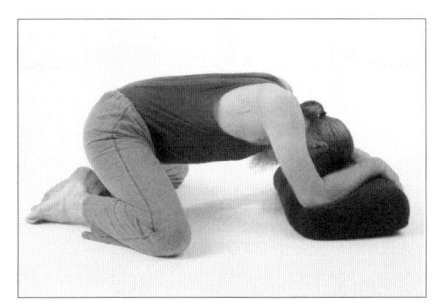

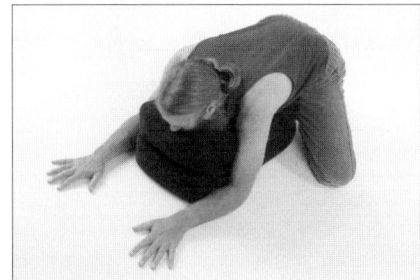

Benefits

Frog is a good stretch for your groin and back. It's also a nice counterpose to Seal and Saddle. Frog relaxes the whole body.

Meridians Stimulated

Frog stimulates the Liver, Kidney, Spleen, and Urinary Bladder meridians and can bring a feeling of overall calm to the body. A harmonious Liver meridian encourages kindness. A harmonious Kidney meridian, with additional support from the Urinary Bladder meridian, puts us in touch with our true essence and inner wisdom, while a healthy Spleen meridian opens us to our creative potential.

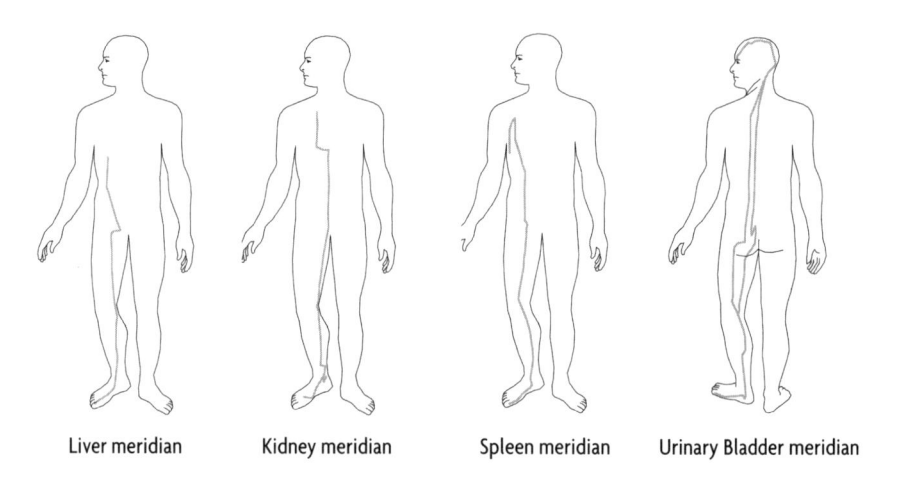

Liver meridian   Kidney meridian   Spleen meridian   Urinary Bladder meridian

Chakras Affected

First (Muladhara), Second (Svadhisthana), and Third (Manipura)

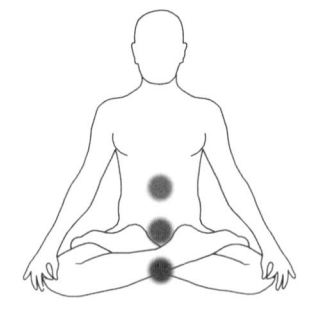

Cautions

If you're not supported in some way, the Frog posture may be stressful for the sacroiliac joint. The unsupported weight of the body will also intensify the groin stretch.

Spinal Twist

Begin on your back with both knees bent and pulled in to your chest. Extend one leg along the floor, letting the bent leg fall over the straight leg toward the floor. Or bend both knees and stack them on top of each other. Don't force the twist; relax and breathe into it. Repeat on the other side.

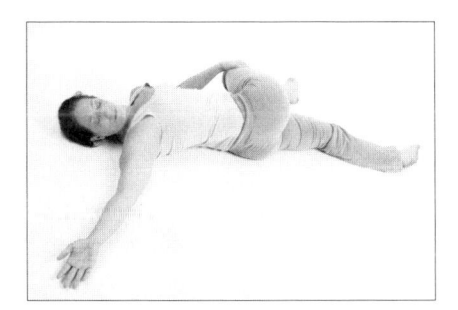

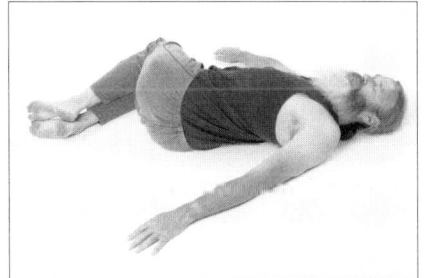

Variations

Feel free to substitute your favorite reclined spinal twist for the one described here. Try using a cushion or blanket under your bent knee and/or under your shoulder if you find either tends to lift off the floor. Muscles relax more easily when they feel supported. By turning your head to one side or another, changing the position of your arms, or sliding your bent knee toward or away from your shoulder, you may feel the stretch in a different way. Don't hesitate to experiment.

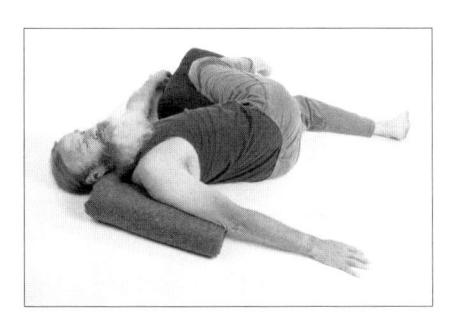

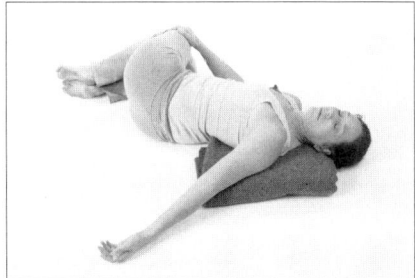

Benefits

Spinal Twist rotates and stretches the whole spine. It also relaxes the mind and opens the heart. Many people feel strong emotions during Spinal Twist, particularly at the end of their practice. You may feel the twist releasing issues that have been held in your first and second chakras, letting them move up into your fourth chakra to come into the light of your heart. This is an excellent pose to do just before Final Relaxation.

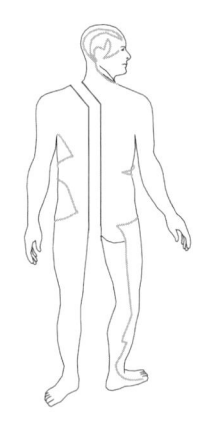

Meridians Stimulated

Spinal Twist primarily stimulates the Gall Bladder Meridian, encouraging us to be courageous and helping us to make reasonable, rational decisions. Spinal Twist may also affect all the meridians in the torso.

Gall Bladder meridian

Chakras Affected

First (Muladhara), Second (Svadhisthana), and Fourth (Anahata)

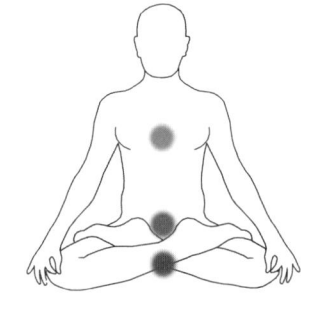

Cautions

Because Spinal Twist is so comfortable for many people, the mind may wander more easily than in more challenging poses. Remember to bring your attention back to your body in a yin, compassionate way.

Final Relaxation

Lie on your back with your palms facing up and your arms and legs spread a comfortable width apart.

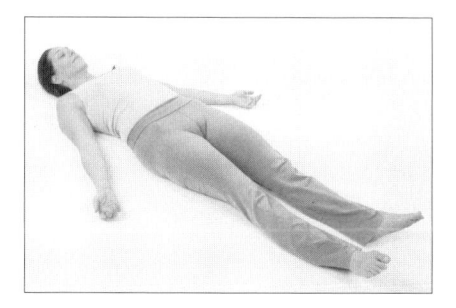

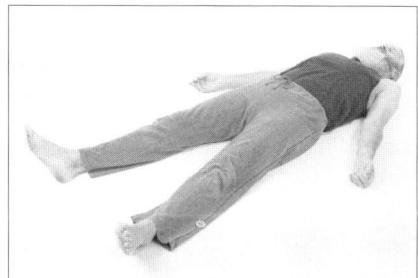

Variations

Assume any position that helps you feel most relaxed. A cushion under the knees can release strain in the lower back. Use a blanket and eye shades to feel cozier.

Benefits

Final Relaxation is a time to bring our awareness to the subtle movement of energy through our bodies, as well as to see more clearly the thought patterns of our minds. In the quiet of this pose, we can reap the benefits of our whole practice.

Meridians Stimulated

By focusing on the flow of energy in our bodies, we encourage the free flow of qi or prana through all the meridians. It is this effortless energy flow within the body that brings calm and harmony to our physical, energetic, and emotional selves.

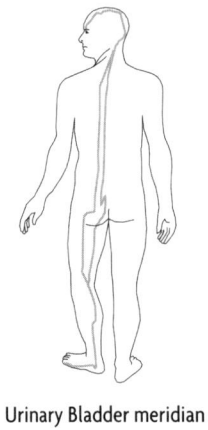

Urinary Bladder meridian 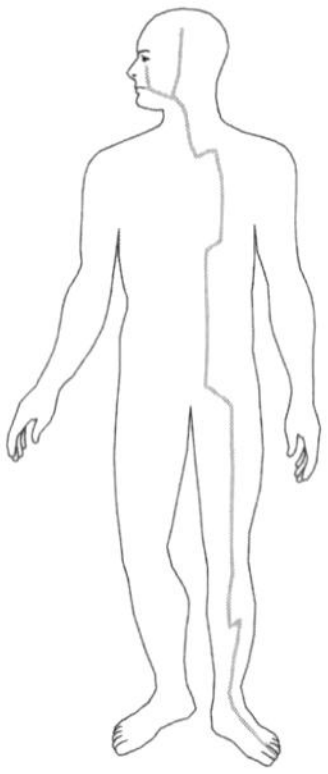 | Stomach meridian 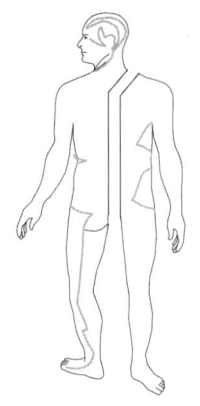 | Gall Bladder meridian

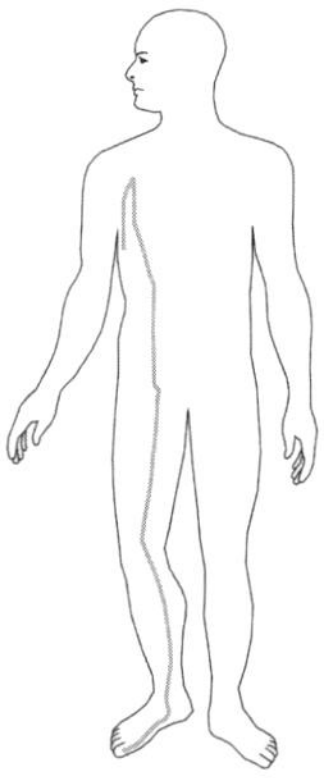

Spleen meridian 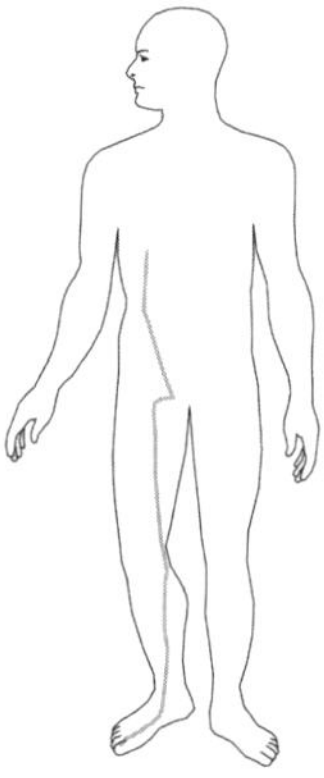 | Liver meridian 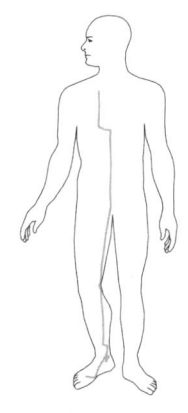 | Kidney meridian

Chakras Affected
Final Relaxation is beneficial for all of our chakras.

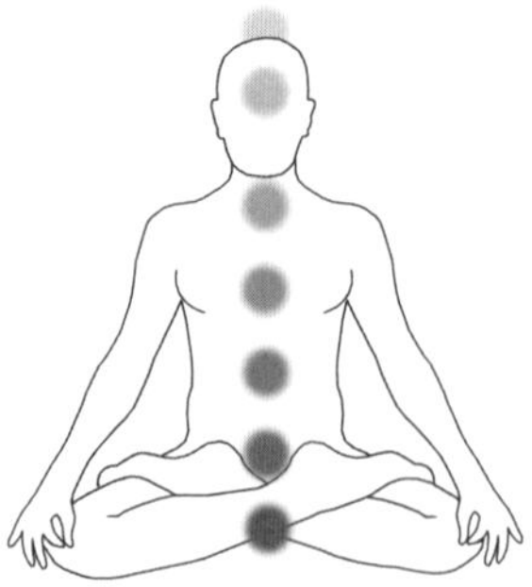

Cautions
Beware of wandering mind, loud snoring.

THE PRACTICE OF MINDFULNESS

Now that I'm in the posture, what do I do? For me, Yin Yoga is a practice of mindfulness. Mindfulness means paying attention and accepting. Being aware. It's not about making judgments as to what's good or bad or whether things are as we think they should be. It's simply about seeing things as they really are. To be mindful we must be willing to drop the filters that our minds often put between us and our experience. We need to let go of the stories we create about ourselves and our lives, the illusions that separate us from our true natures and from one another. Our minds are often reluctant to accept the experiences of our lives without judging each experience as good or bad, something we want more of or something we don't ever want again. It is from this kind of attachment, this clinging or aversion, that much of our suffering arises.

In mindfulness practice we bring our attention to whatever is happening in the present moment. When we walk, we know we're walking. We don't worry about where we're going or if we would rather be taking a bus, we simply turn our attention to the fact that we're walking. If our feet get tired, we simply notice that they're tired; we don't wish it otherwise. Of course, if they get too tired, perhaps we'll choose to sit for a while and then, without judgment, we'll just notice that we're sitting. In my Yin Yoga practice, as in my meditation, I try to practice mindfulness.

I find that I use mindfulness in my Yin practice in two different ways: mindfulness of my breath and mindfulness of specific parts of my body where I feel intense sensations, those places where energy feels stuck. I start in each posture with mindfulness of breath. Meditation practices offer many tools to help bring attention to the breath. It would be fine to use any tools that you're comfortable with in your Yin Yoga practice. I most deeply connect with the very simple practices taught by the wonderful teacher Thich Nhat Hanh. When I meditate or assume a Yin posture, I simply say to myself on my inhale,

Breathing in, I know that I'm breathing in.

And on my exhale,

Breathing out, I know that I'm breathing out.

By bringing this simple awareness to the breath, without judgment or control, without striving to make it any different, the breath will naturally lengthen and deepen. The mind will begin to quiet, to be more at peace. By just being aware of the breath, without the need to change things, we can find real joy in the simple practice of breathing. Joy in just being alive right where we always are—in the present moment. This is the yin way. Instead of making an effort to control the breath, or even our thoughts, we can just watch and accept with compassion. Our breath will calm and our mind will still.

For me, mindfulness is about simple joy—the joy of breathing, the joy of being alive, the joy of being just who we are, the joy of this perfect present moment. When I really bring my attention to something as simple as breathing, I begin to feel a magic leading me to become still and present.

This is another mantra by Thich Nhat Hanh that I often use:

On the inhale,

> *Breathing in, I calm myself.*

On the exhale,

> *Breathing out, I smile.*

On the inhale,

> *Breathing in, I know that this is the perfect moment.*

On the exhale,

> *Breathing out, I know that this is the only moment.*

Of course, in any practice of stillness, such as Yin Yoga or meditation, our minds will wander. This is true for every normal person (if you are already totally enlightened please skip the next section). But when your mind wanders and you begin to think or judge or consider what to have for breakfast, the important thing is to bring your mind back to your breath, to the present moment, in a yin way, in a way that holds no blame or judgment, in a compassionate way.

When you are in a Yin pose you'll often experience an intensity or feeling—a tension or holding in some part of your body. I most often feel Yin postures in my lower back or hips. When I do, I find it helpful to focus my attention on the area of intensity. First I try to look at what's really going on there. I ask myself, *Is the sensation I'm feeling something that seems to be good for me? Is it a nice stretch of my muscle and connective tissue or a gentle healthy compression, or am I in the pose too deeply and is what I'm feeling a signal to modify my position or come out of the pose?* Even when I bring my full attention to my sensation, it's not always easy to tell. This is a question that all practitioners of any form of yoga must answer for themselves in their own practices. If your breath feels restricted or raggedy in the pose, it is a sign that you are in the pose too deeply. If you are not able to breathe smoothly and evenly then the pose is not beneficial to you in the way that you're practicing it. If you ever feel that the way you're practicing a pose may cause you injury, I would urge you to pay attention to that feeling and to stop doing whatever is causing you to feel that way. It's important in any yoga to understand that all of our bodies are different; what works and is beneficial for one person will be harmful for someone else. Each body is also different from day to day and hour to hour. A posture that was great for you yesterday may be too much for you today. Not all yoga postures are right for everyone. With attention and practice, you'll become more skillful at knowing which postures and modifications are best for you.

However, if the intensity feels as though it's stretching and bringing healing energy to the area, it's a good practice to just joyfully notice what's happening. I like to use a mantra such as the following:

Breathing in, I notice that I'm tense in the lower back
[substitute any body part where you might be holding tension].
Breathing out, I smile at my lower back.

I sometimes use what you might call a more proactive mantra if I feel stuck or challenged in a particular area. I often use this one in Seal or Saddle:

Breathing in, I feel tension in my lower back.
Breathing out, I let go of that tension.

Mantras are powerful tools for focusing your attention and I invite you to create your own. It's your body and your practice; why not have your own mantra?

Bringing attention and breath to any aspect of ourselves, emotional, energetic, or physical, will create space for change. You will feel things let go, relax, become easier, not because you demanded it but simply because you allowed it. By nourishing a yin attitude of compassionate acceptance, we allow the wisdom of our bodies to be heard.

THE PRACTICE OF LOVING KINDNESS

I want to discuss a very important practice that I think fits naturally with Yin Yoga. It's called the practice of Loving Kindness, or in the ancient Pali language, Metta.

For me, the heart of Yin Yoga is Loving Kindness, compassion and acceptance—the energy of the Mother.

Loving Kindness is a state of unconditional love, a place from which we can give our love and best wishes to ourselves and to others without judgment or expectation. In Metta practice we see things as they are. We see ourselves and others clearly, with acceptance, our feelings of separation falling away. From the practice of Loving Kindness develops compassion, sympathetic joy, and equanimity. Although Loving Kindness and compassion are subtly different concepts and are often practiced separately, because I practice them as one practice, I present them here in that way. We direct this Loving Kindness and compassion at ourselves as we do the practice, but we also know somewhere within ourselves that any Loving Kindness and compassion we show to ourselves, we show to all beings. If we understand the Taoist way of seeing the world, we know that we are all connected; the same qi flows through us all. Metta is a way of practicing this knowing.

In Metta practice, we use a repeated phrase or mantra to ask for health and peace. The practice always begins by asking for health and peace for yourself. These are the Metta phrases I use most often:

> *May I be free of fear and harm*
> *May I be happy just the way I am*
> *May I be at peace with whatever comes*
> *And may I learn to live gently in the softness of my own heart.*

There are many other variations by other practitioners, some of which are found in the books by Sharon Salzburg, Jack Kornfield, or Thich Nhat Hanh listed in the resources section at the end of this book. You can also use any words that have meaning for you.

It is good to repeat this mantra until you can feel compassion, acceptance, and forgiveness for yourself. This can happen right away or it can take much longer. It's important to remember that this isn't a selfish practice. We know that when we bring happiness to ourselves, we make the whole world happier. Only when we feel compassion for ourselves, can we start to take that compassion out into the world.

The next step is to change the wording slightly by asking that someone close to us also receive the benefits of our desire to end his or her suffering. You might say something like this:

> *May all my family be free of fear and harm*
> *May they be happy just as they are*
> *May they be at peace with whatever comes*
> *And may they live gently in the softness of their own hearts.*

You can substitute your friends or coworkers, anyone you particularly care about.

When you feel that your Loving Kindness and compassion flows easily to the people you have included in your mantra, you can begin to broaden the circle of compassion to someone you might feel neutral about, substituting that person's name in the mantra. Finally, when you feel ready, you can include someone who is a challenge to you, someone toward whom you have difficulty feeling compassion. This may take some work. You can finish your practice by including all beings. It is also a wonderful practice to skip right to the last part, asking:

May all beings be free of fear and harm
May we all be happy just the way we are
May we all be at peace with whatever comes
And may we all live gently in the softness of our own hearts.

It's important to remember that the practice begins with a feeling of Loving Kindness and compassion for ourselves, including the acceptance that we may have real problems feeling this way toward some people in the world. It's a practice; all we really need to do is practice with intention.

USING THE YIN YOGA KIT TO DESIGN YOUR PERSONAL PRACTICE

Along with this book, you will find an audio CD and a set of fourteen posture cards in your *Yin Yoga Kit*. These materials have been included to help you develop a personal practice that works for you. To help you get started, I lead you verbally through a ten-posture sequence on the CD, speaking as I do when I'm teaching a Yin Yoga class. But it is my hope that over time you will begin to design your own practice—doing the postures in whatever sequence feels best on any given day. You can use the Yin Yoga cards to help you plan each practice. If you are a yoga teacher, you can use the cards to more easily plan your classes.

How to Use the Yin Yoga CD

The audio CD that has been included in *The Yin Yoga Kit* contains thirteen tracks. On the first track I've outlined some things that I think are important to consider when starting your Yin Yoga practice. On tracks 2 through 11 I'll lead you through a practice of ten postures. Each posture will be held for five minutes followed by a one-minute rest period. The entire sequence lasts approximately one hour. Track 12 is a Metta meditation, or prayer of Loving Kindness, that I recite during or after my own practice (as discussed in the chapter on Loving Kindness). Track 13 is designed as a timer for you to use when practicing your own sequence of postures.

During the ten-posture sample practice part of the CD, I'll talk about each posture itself; possible variations to the posture, including props you might want to use; and ways in which the posture may affect your meridians and chakras. I'll also discuss the practice of mindfulness and attention to the breath and body, and I'll introduce the use of mantras as a way of focusing attention. As often as time allows I'll leave periods of silence, for it is in silence that I believe the real meditative practice of Yin Yoga may be most easily experienced. During the rest periods between postures, I'll invite you to bring your attention to your body in order to feel any physical, emotional, or energetic sensations that may have arisen from practicing. I've chosen to use a gentle drone sound during the rest periods.

Before you turn on the CD to begin following the sample practice, you may find it helpful to get out your Yin Yoga cards and arrange them in the order in which I introduce the postures. You can use the pictures on the cards for guidance while you practice. The sequence is listed below.

Track 1: Introduction
Track 2: Half Butterfly
Track 3: Half Butterfly side II
Track 4: Seal
Track 5: Frog
Track 6: Shoelace
Track 7: Shoelace side II
Track 8: Saddle

Using the Yin Yoga Kit to Design Your Personal Practice • 81

Track 9: Spinal Twist
Track 10: Spinal Twist side II
Track 11: Resting Pose

On track 11 I've included Resting Pose rather than Final Relaxation because I wanted to give you a guided practice for relaxing the important pelvic muscle group, the iliopsoas (see more on the iliopsoas in Part 3 on page 92). Resting Pose is also a good way to begin a practice, particularly if you feel tight or restricted in your pelvic area.

Because of time constraints, I haven't been able to include on the CD all the postures that I've presented in the book and card set, but the ten I include represent the full range of motion available to the spine and hips. The practice information I've given on the CD should prove helpful for all the postures. Because each posture is on a separate track, if you have a programmable CD player, you can rearrange the tracks in any order you like or skip some altogether.

When you're ready to move on to designing your own sequence of postures, without my narration, you can use track 13 to time your practice. It begins with one ring of a bell, signaling the beginning of the first posture. After five minutes the bell rings twice, signaling the end of the posture and the beginning of the rest period. After the one-minute rest period the bell sounds three times. If your CD player has a repeat function you can set it to repeat track 13. Then, while using the cards to remind you of your chosen practice sequence, you can relax and let the bells tell you when it is time to change postures.

You can also program your player to insert track 13 anywhere in the CD so you can choose to do one of the postures on the cards in place of, or in addition to, any of the postures on the CD. You may choose to go into Resting Pose first and follow the guided practice with your own Final Relaxation. In that case you could program track 13 after your last posture, using it to time your Final Relaxation, followed by track 12, the closing meditation. Not all postures work for everyone, so feel free to substitute anywhere you see fit. This is your practice.

Although I've chosen to hold each pose for five minutes, you may find this time period to be too long or too short. You may also find that some of the postures aren't beneficial for you right now. Please pay attention to what *you* feel and let yourself be guided by your own experience. Only go as deeply and stay as long in any pose as feels right to you. When you listen to your body, you'll know what it really needs. Many people like to play music during the poses. If you find that music helps you relax and deepens your practice, that's fine. I would encourage you, however, to be sure that the music is helping to lead you deeper and not just leading you away from things you may find difficult.

Yin Yoga is a very personal practice. Its true benefits come from going deeply within yourself and being mindful of what's true for you. This CD is designed to help you get started in your practice but is not intended to *become* your practice. It's my hope that you'll use the CD a few times, then, with help from the card set, you'll let your body, breath, mind, and heart guide you in developing your own practice.

How to Use the Yin Yoga Cards

The Yin Yoga cards are intended to help you design your own practice. Follow the three easy steps below when deciding upon a sequence of postures.

Step One: Decide how long you want to practice and how long you want to hold each posture. For many people five minutes per pose feels right, but let your body guide you. Now you need to determine how many poses you will have time for. For example: Say you intend to practice for one hour and you want to hold each pose the suggested time of five minutes per pose. Allowing one minute to rest between poses, each pose will take about six minutes; you'll therefore have time for ten poses. Remember that some postures, such as Half Butterfly or Spinal Twist, must be done first on one side, and then

Using the Yin Yoga Kit to Design Your Personal Practice • 83

repeated for a second five minutes on the other side. So in terms of the total time allotted, each side counts as one five-minute posture. You will soon discover how much time it actually takes you to transition from pose to pose and how much rest you like to take between poses. You may also find that you like to meditate or do some breathing exercise *(pranayama)* before or after your practice.

Step Two: Choose cards from the deck that you feel would be most beneficial for you at that moment. For example: If you are feeling stiff in the lower back, you might start with Half Butterfly rather than Forward Bend, which is a more demanding posture. If you are feeling sluggish, you might want to do Seal early in your practice, as back bends tend to energize us. I often begin my practices in Resting Pose and end in meditation. You will soon learn which poses work best for your body at any given time.

You may find that alternating between forward bends and back bends, wider-legged poses, and poses with legs closer together adds a greater balance to your practice. I have discussed sequencing further in Part 3 in the section on the range of motion in the hips and spine. I suggest planning your practice in a way that brings you balance and takes your hips and spine through their full range of motion.

Step Three: Arrange the cards you've chosen in the order you want to practice the postures and keep them next to your mat for easy reference. Program your CD player to repeat track 13 or place a regular kitchen timer or a watch with a built-in timer near your mat. Special meditation timers are also available and have a more soothing tone. If you're using a timer, set it for the length of time that you have decided to hold each pose. Then start the timer (or start track 13 on your CD player) and take the first pose. Now forget about the timer and what you're going to do next and just be in the pose. Breathe. Soften. Be in the present moment. When the timer rings, just come slowly out of the pose, relax on your back or your belly, and then refer to the next card you've chosen to guide you into your next posture. Resting between poses helps you feel the effects of each pose and helps sharpen your awareness of the movement of qi throughout your body. Although Yin Yoga is a form of meditation, I would suggest allowing time for sitting meditation before or after your practice whenever possible.

By using a timer and planning each practice session with the Yin Yoga cards, you can more easily let your mind relax during your practice, without having to consider how much time you have left in the current posture or which postures you want to do next. It is important, however, to listen to your body—if at any time the practice you planned for yourself no longer feels right, honor that feeling and modify the practice to follow your inner wisdom.

At the top of each card I have suggested some ways in which the pose may affect you physically, energetically, or emotionally. You will find these suggestions discussed in far more detail in the descriptions for each posture in the book, as well as in the chapters on the meridians and chakras. These chapters outline the potential emotional and energetic influences of each meridian and chakra stimulated by Yin Yoga postures.

I have included two pictures of the featured pose per card, showing how the posture might look for people with different ranges of motion. Whether you are hypermobile and can go into poses very deeply or you meet your edge more quickly in the pose, makes no difference in how the pose affects you physically or energetically. Our bodies are all different and it is our anatomical differences that ultimately affect the form of our yoga poses. Let go of any ideas about how you should look or how deep your pose should be, and just gratefully accept where you are right now.

The Use of Props

Yin Yoga relaxes the muscles (the more yang parts of the body) so that the connective tissue and bones (the more yin parts) can receive our attention. Muscles are able to relax more easily when they feel safe and supported. The use of props can be a great help in providing a sense of comfort and support.

Try using cushions or bolsters under any part of the body that feels as though it's hanging unsupported. For many people, an example of this would be putting a cushion under the bent knee or knees in Half or Full Butterfly. Some people like to stack cushions on which to rest their head and chest in any forward bend. In Spinal Twist, supporting the shoulder or knee can allow more relaxation and a deeper experience. A rolled-up towel, or the kind of foam noodle people use in their swimming pools, works well for support under the ankles or behind the knees in Saddle.

It's important to remember, however, that in order for Yin Yoga to be most effective it needs to bring some gentle tension to the parts of the body that it specifically targets. For example, if we use cushions to support the lower back in Saddle, the posture becomes more of a restorative one. Although as a restorative posture it can have great benefits, it no longer affects the sacrum and lumbar spine in the same way that Saddle does.

These are just examples of what works for some people. You will find more suggestions for props in the section that describes each posture. Experiment! It's your practice and your body (and probably your cushions), so use props wherever your body asks for them.

Part 3

Anatomy and Yin Yoga

THE CONNECTIVE TISSUE

Because we hold postures for extended periods in Yin Yoga and move deeply into them while allowing our muscles to relax, the postures are able to put gentle corrective tension on our deep connective tissue. Connective tissue runs throughout the body in many forms. Some of the most familiar are fascia, tendons, and ligaments. The connective tissue forms a web, which essentially holds the body together and allows the muscles and organs to function properly. Yin Yoga is concerned mainly with the ligaments, the tissue that holds bone to bone, encapsulates each joint, and contains the lubricating sinovial fluid.

The spinal column is wrapped tightly with approximately seven layer of connective tissue. Ligaments hold the pelvis to the spine and the thigh bones (femurs) to the pelvis. Much of the fluidity of movement and the range of motion in the body is dependant upon healthy connective tissue. As with muscles, connective tissue begins to lose its range of motion if it's not used. The ligaments can begin to dry and contract with age, and this degeneration is accelerated by our sedentary lifestyles. We often see the effects of compromised connective tissue in older people as the connective tissue around the spine shrinks, affecting the spinal disks

THE CONNECTIVE TISSUE • 89

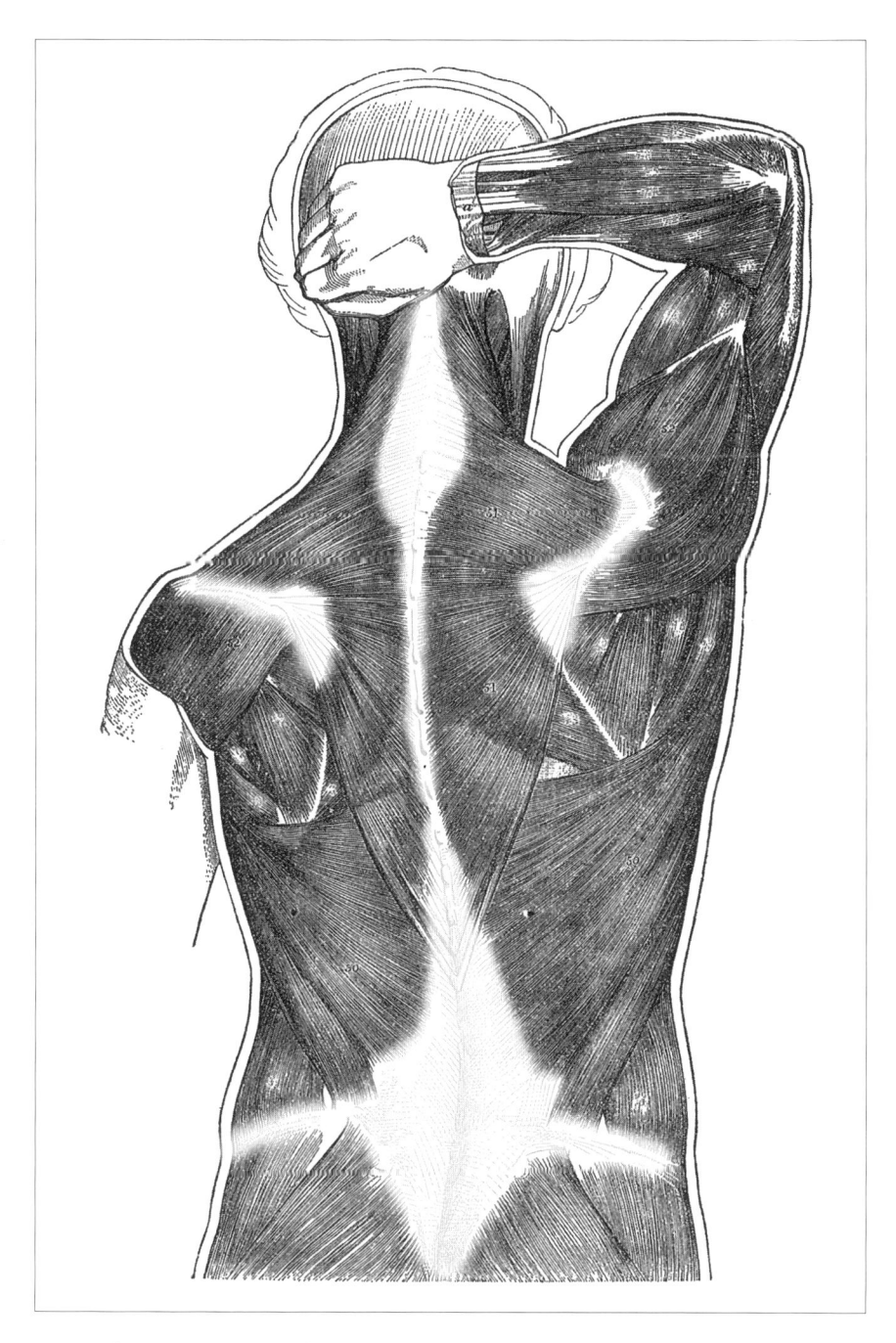

The connective tissue holds the body together. In this illustration the lighter areas show the connective tissue surrounding the pelvis, spine, and shoulder joints.

and vertebrae, which causes pain and immobility. The disks themselves, which consist largely of connective tissue, can also dry up and lose their resiliency if we cease to use the full range of motion available to our spines.

According to Roger Jahnke, director of the Institute of Integral Qigong and Tai Chi, the origins of connective-tissue-transforming practice in the qigong (or Chinese yoga) tradition extend back into prehistory. Shamanic dances and practices for merging with nature included connective-tissue-focused practices. The most widely known version is known as Yi Jin Jing—connective-tissue-transforming classic practice.

The Taoists and martial artists continued this kind of practice for centuries and it became a foundation in medical and healing qigong. The most widely circulated story of the origin of Yi Jin Jing, probably more of a myth given the history already noted, is that Bodhidharma, the originator of Zen (Chan Buddhism), brought the practices to China from India around 500 CE.

The integration of body movement, breathing practice, deep meditative relaxation, and self-applied massage with a focus on the connective tissue is a form of qigong with roots that may extend 5000 or even 10,000 years into shamanic prehistory.

Following in this connective-tissue-transforming tradition, Yin Yoga primarily targets the connective tissue of the lower back (the lumbar spine), the pelvis, and the hip sockets (femur and acetabulum). By relaxing the muscles around the joints in these areas, we place gentle, controlled stress on the connective tissue and bones. Because connective tissue is both much drier and less flexible than muscle, it doesn't respond to the type of stress that muscle most appreciates. Muscle likes yang exercise—active and repetitive movement—while the connective tissue needs a more yin style of movement—gentle and controlled, with longer holds. When we hold a posture without striving, we apply a gentle tension to the connective tissue that begins to counteract the effects of aging and gravity. In this way, through Yin Yoga, we can preserve and even increase the range of motion in our joints.

THE SACRUM AND THE LUMBAR SPINE

A very important joint in Yin Yoga, and in our everyday life, is the joint between the sacrum (the triangular bone at the base of the spine) and the ilium (the pelvis). This is commonly known as the sacroiliac, or S.I., joint. The comfort of the lower back and the whole pelvic region relies heavily on the proper alignment of this joint. In its natural healthy position, the sacrum should tilt forward at the top, following the natural curve of the lower back (the lumbar curve). Because we spend so much time sitting in chairs with our lower backs slouched, our sacrum starts to tilt backward, so that it no longer fits easily into its natural home in the ilium. This postural misalignment is a major cause of lower-back pain and immobility. As the sacrum tilts back, the lumbar spine also flattens and loses much of its strength and resiliency. As we get older, the flattening of the sacrum and lumbar curve can lead to strain in the back and pelvis and even contribute to the degeneration of the vertebrae and intervertebral disks.

It's important in Yin practice to maintain a forward tilt to the sacrum.

In postures involving forward bends, it's often necessary to use a cushion under the sitz bones to maintain the proper tilt and to allow gravity to help us stay more comfortably in the pose. If you have trouble leaning forward, you can bend your knees, which releases the hamstrings and allows the pelvis to tilt forward more easily. It's also helpful to begin the forward bend with a straight back, which allows the powerful back muscles to help pull the pelvis and sacrum forward.

In Seal it's best not to try to tuck your tailbone under, as that flattens the lower back and sacrum, but rather to let the sacrum tilt forward and the spine curve naturally with no effort. Saddle is a very powerful pose for the health of the lumbar and sacral area. The important thing to remember about Saddle is to be gentle—don't push too hard; have patience.

Relaxing the Iliopsoas

Two muscles, the psoas major and the iliacus, together make up the iliopsoas muscle group. The iliopsoas connects the spine, the pelvis, and the legs, and is therefore very important in the stabilization of the whole pelvic region.

The psoas muscle originates at the lowest thoracic vertebra (T-12) and all five of the lumbar vertebrae (L-1 through L-5). The iliacus muscle originates at the upper inside surface and crest of the iliac bone—the wide fan-shaped bone that you can feel at your upper forward hip or pelvis. The two muscles join and run together over the front of the hip socket and attach to the femur (thigh) bone on the inside of the leg at the lesser trochanter (see labeled illustration of the femur on page 97).

The iliopsoas is a hip flexor. In other words, it helps to bring the leg forward when we walk. Although it does not initiate the movement of walking, the iliopsoas contracts as our weight shifts forward, acting almost like a rope or pendulum to help the leg swing freely forward. Then, in its healthy relaxed state, the iliopsoas releases, allowing the leg to swing smoothly back. At the same time, because of its multiple

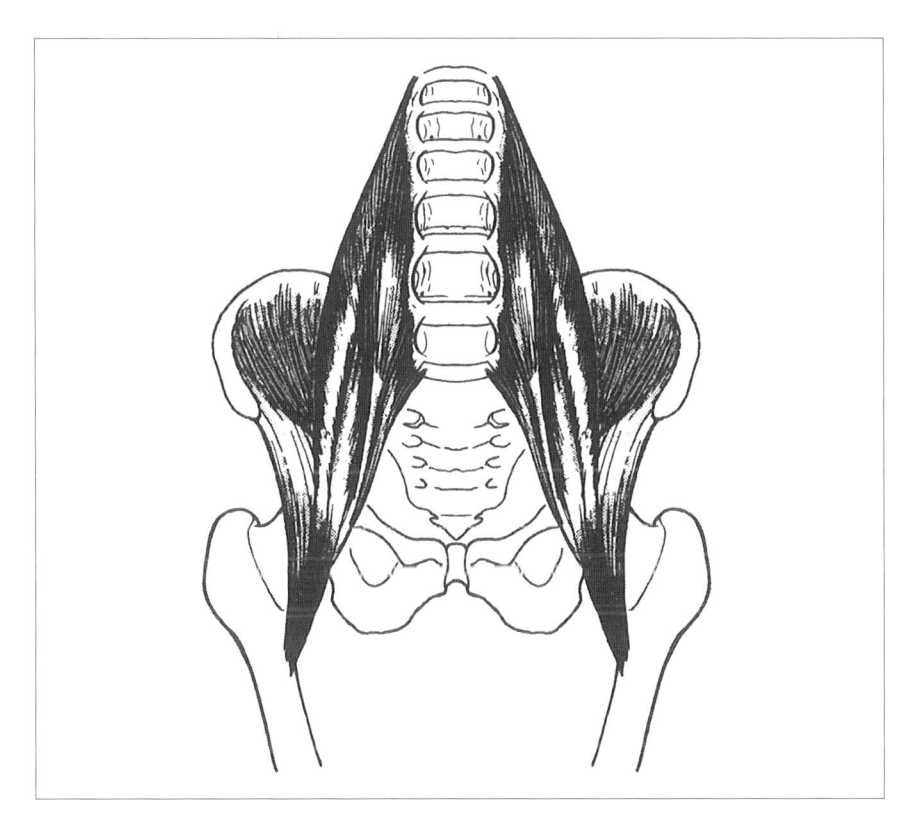

The muscles in the iliopsoas muscle group
are the only muscles that connect the spine, pelvis, and legs.

attachments, it helps to maintain the stability and alignment of the hips and lower spine.

The iliopsoas, however, is very susceptible to holding tension and not releasing completely when its job is done. This chronic tension can be triggered by long periods of sitting or driving. The muscle group is also closely connected with our ancient fight-or-flight response. When we're in a state of danger, the iliopsoas prepares itself to respond by tensing and contracting. When the danger passes the muscle should release. It's very common, however, for the iliopsoas to lose its ability to relax. I believe that it remains in a constant state of tension because we live in a world where we often feel helpless and unsafe. When the iliopsoas doesn't release properly, the tension can put a strain on the whole pelvic area, moving it out of alignment and causing stiffness and discomfort in the lower back, pelvis, and hips, as well as pain in the groin and abdomen. Chronic iliopsoas tension is also believed to be a contributing factor in such conditions as prostatitis and chronic pelvic pain.

Practicing Resting Pose is a very good way to release the iliopsoas muscles. On the audio CD I've presented a guided meditation on releasing tension in the iliopsoas, which I've found to be an effective way to begin to drop the tension that so many of us carry in this very important muscle group.

TENSION AND COMPRESSION

Understanding is the foundation of compassion.
THICH NHAT HANH

A lot of our suffering in yoga comes when we think that our yoga practice should be just like the practice of the person next to us in class. We embrace our yang need to strive and change, while disregarding our yin nature of acceptance. We all come to points of restriction in the body as we reach the end of our range of motion. By understanding what causes these restrictions we can bring more self-acceptance into our practice.

There are two factors that determine our range of motion and the way we look in any yoga posture:

The first is the restriction that comes when our muscles won't stretch any further. This is a tensile restriction and is very familiar to any yoga practitioner. If we stand up and bend over to touch our toes, most people, especially before they're warmed up, will be stopped from going any further when their hamstrings (the muscles at the back of thigh) will no longer stretch. As we warm up or continue to practice yoga, our hamstrings will loosen and allow our forward bend to go deeper. This is a muscular type of restriction and because the muscles have a yang nature, they love movement. If we move them in a yang way, striving to change them, they will respond by changing and becoming longer and more flexible. We can work hard to get past our muscular or tensile restrictions, but at some point, no matter how hard we work, we just won't get any further. This is a point at which many people get frustrated and discouraged. They know that they're working as hard as anyone in the class, but they still can't sit in Full Lotus. This might not be so bad, but the guy next to them, who hardly ever comes to class, calmly puts down his café latte, goes into Full Lotus, and begins to complain to his neighbor about how stiff he's feeling today.

All the stretching in the world will only take you so far. In everyone's body and in every posture there comes a point where the restriction we experience is no longer caused by our muscles. When we have worked through our muscular or tensile restriction, we reach a point where our joints come into compression. In compression, either the bones hit each other (as essentially happens when we fully straighten our elbow) or tissue becomes pinched between the bones (as happens in most other joints). This compressive restriction occurs at the more yin parts of our bodies, the bones and connective tissue. Although hard work and striving can change the tensile restrictions in our muscles, when we come into compressive restriction at the level of the bones we need to accept ourselves as we are.

Different people reach compressive restriction at different points. That's because we're all unique. Our heads are shaped differently from one another's, we have longer legs or smaller feet or bigger hands than the person sitting next to us. These differences are a reflection of the different shapes of our bones. When we understand that the way our yoga postures look and feel to us is ultimately dependent upon when our bones come into compressive restriction, it becomes obvious that any differences we have at the skeletal level will make a big difference to our practice. In Yin Yoga postures, variations in the shape and size of our femurs, or thigh bones, have the biggest effect upon our range of motion.

Tension and Compression • 97

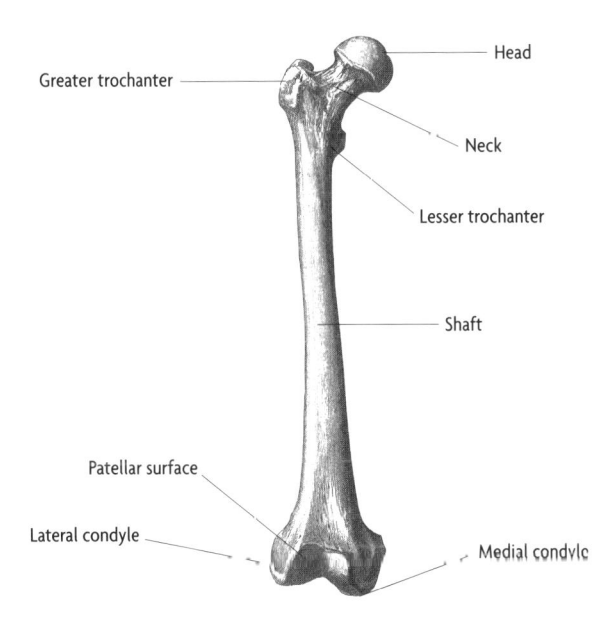

Greater trochanter
Head
Neck
Lesser trochanter
Shaft
Patellar surface
Lateral condyle
Medial condyle

The human femur

If you examine human femurs from a number of skeletons you'll see marked differences among them. There will be variations in the ways that the heads of the femurs line up with the knees or in the angles of the femur heads in relation to the shafts or in the neck lengths of the various femurs. You can see some of these differences in the picture of human femurs below.

Human femurs showing natural variations in length and width, torque, head angles, and length of necks.

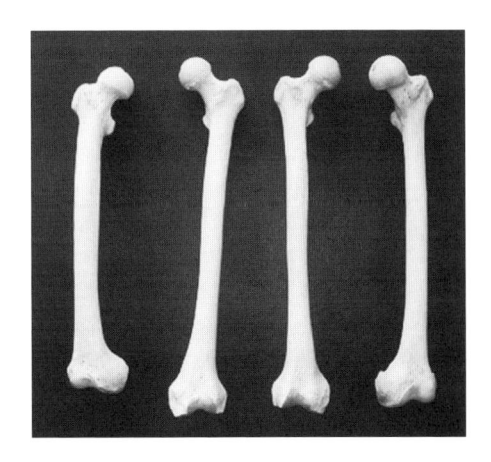

We are not at all surprised when we see someone who obviously has longer femurs than we do; we expect to see those differences. What we often don't think about is the differences that we can't see in the shapes of the bones. We know that a person with long leg bones or arm bones can probably reach things from a higher shelf than we can. Most of us don't believe that if we worked harder we could reach as high as the person with longer arms and legs. We generally just accept that the other person is taller and get on with our lives. However, differences in such areas as the length of the neck of the femur, a difference we can't ordinarily see, can make a big difference in our range of motion. Notice how the second femur in the picture on page 97 has more distance between the head (the round knob at the upper end) and the shaft (or long part of the bone) than the femur to its left. We can describe this difference by saying that the second femur has a longer neck than the first. As we abduct our femurs when we spread our legs in postures like Dragonfly (see page 63), the greater trochanter (the bump on the outside of the femur where certain muscles attach) compresses tissue between itself and the pelvis. It is this compressive restriction that ultimately stops our legs from widening (abducting) any further. How soon this compression occurs depends in part on the length of the neck of the femur. All other factors being equal, the shorter the neck of the femur, the sooner compressive restriction will occur. When we accept that we have as many differences in the shape and length of the necks of our femurs as we do in the shape and size of our heads (or the necks they sits on), it makes perfect sense that our Dragonfly will look different than the Dragonfly of the person next to us.

Another place that differences occur between one person's femur and another's is in the twist of the shaft, in other words, in the relationship between the patella (or knee) and the angle of the head of the femur as it fits into the hip socket (acetabulum). In the picture at the top of page 99 you can see that when the surfaces behind where the kneecap sits (the lateral and medial condyles) are sitting on the floor parallel to one another, the angle of the neck of each femur can be very different. These variations in angle can make a big difference in how much

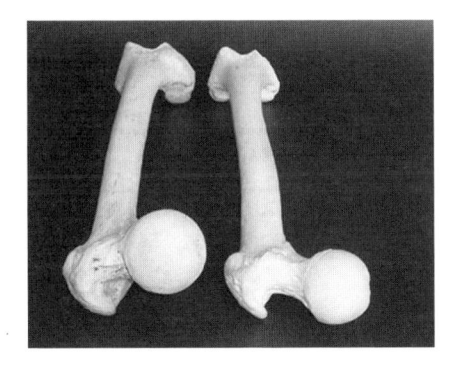

Variations in the twist of the femur shaft affect rotation.

a person's legs can rotate (turn in or out) before they come to a point of compressive restriction. One person may rotate externally very easily but be much more restricted when trying to internally rotate, while another person may have the opposite experience.

The picture below shows a substantial difference between the two femurs in the angle between the neck of the femur and the shaft. You can see that the neck angle of the femur on the left is wider than the angle on the right-hand femur. This means that the femur on the left would be able to abduct (spread apart) further than the one on the right before compression would occur between the greater trochanter (at the lower end in the picture as the femurs are shown upside down) and the hip socket.

So there are two kinds of restriction that control our range of motion: tensile restriction in the muscles and compressive restriction in the bones. Once we have worked through the muscular restrictions we encounter in a posture, we will eventually come into compressive

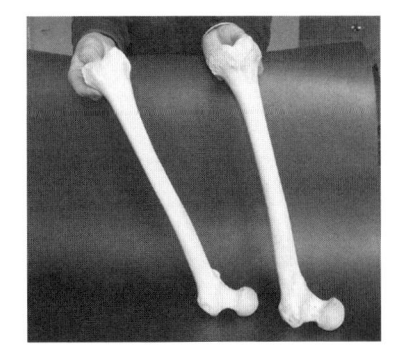

Variations in the angle between neck and shaft affect abduction.

restriction at the bones. The practice that helped us move through our muscular restriction will not help us through compressive restriction. The physical differences that produce compressive restriction are in our bones and nothing short of surgery or braces will safely change them. When we recognize that we are in compressive restriction, we need to shift from an attitude of striving to one of acceptance.

It is not always easy to tell if the restriction we feel is produced by tension or compression. Often tensile restriction feels like a nice stretch. We feel it in the backs of our joints, or away from the direction in which the joint is being moved, as the muscles lengthen. We are more apt to feel compression on the front side of the joint, or toward the direction in which the joint is being moved, as tissue becomes pinched. There is nothing wrong with bringing the joints into compression, as long as it is done with attention and in a yin way, without the expectation of change. It is not a good idea to move forcefully into compression. This is the yang way and though forceful movement is just what yang muscle needs, it is not what yin tissue needs. Much of Yin Yoga is, in fact, about compression. We let the muscles relax so that we can bring beneficial attention to the connective tissue, keeping it healthy and promoting the flow of qi—where attention goes, qi flows. Compression, on the other hand, is not necessarily good for nerves. If you feel a kind of electric sensation in any posture that feels as though you could be pinching a nerve, it is best to come out of the posture or modify your position.

Both yin and yang are always present and necessary. We create suffering for ourselves when we approach our yin self in a yang way, when we think that those parts of ourselves that we can't change need to be changed, when we think that we're not good enough the way we are.

> *Each of you is perfect the way you are . . .*
> *and you can use a little improvement.*
> — SUZUKI ROSHI,
> FROM *TO SHINE ONE CORNER*

MOVEMENT IN THE HIPS AND SPINE

Every joint of the body moves in its own specific way. Yin Yoga focuses primarily on the joints of the hips and the lower spine. By understanding a little about how these joints move, we can more easily decide which Yin postures we want to include in any given practice and why.

Movement in the Hip Joints

The hip joints consist of the femurs (thigh bones) and the pelvis. The head of the femur has a smooth surface that rests in an equally smooth indentation, or socket, in the pelvis called the acetabulum. The hip joint is held together in part by muscles but primarily by strong bands of connective tissue. This connective tissue, which holds bone to bone at the joints, is called ligament.

A number of muscles that originate at the spine or in the pelvic area and attach at the femur or knee are responsible for the movement of the femurs in relation to the pelvis. These muscles move the femur, and therefore the entire leg, in the following six different directions. (All other movements are just combinations of these six.)

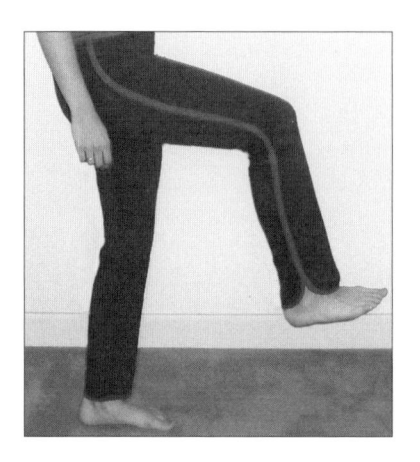

1. Flexion: the thigh moves toward the chest

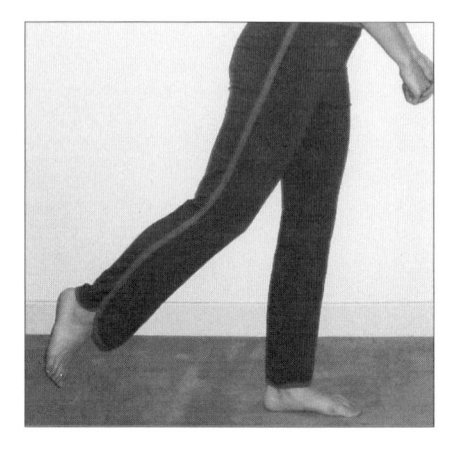

2. Extension: the thigh moves away from the chest

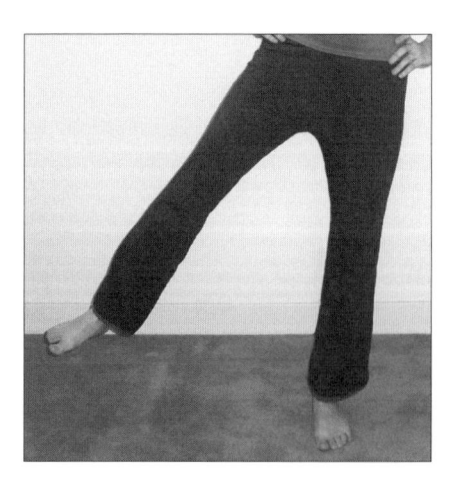

3. Abduction: the leg widens away from the midline of the body, i.e., the right leg moves toward the right and vice versa

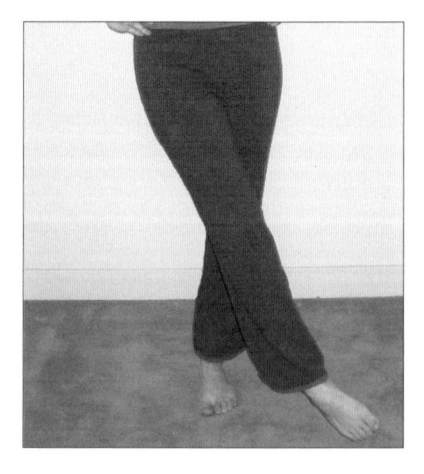

4. Adduction: the leg moves toward or through the midline of the body, i.e., the right leg moves to the left and vice versa

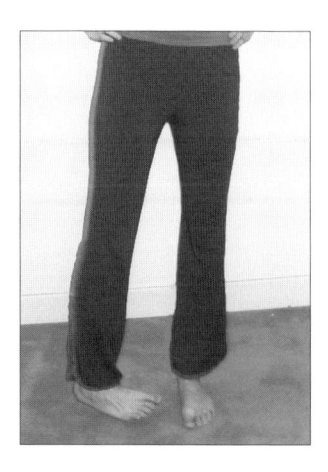

5. Internal Rotation: the right leg rotates to the left or vice versa, i.e., the right leg rotates counter clockwise as you look down on it

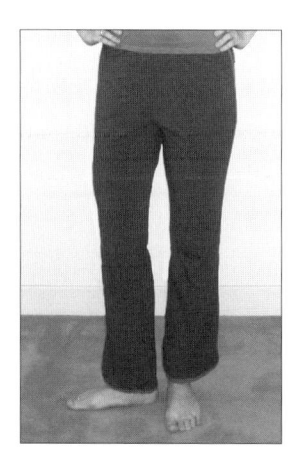

6. External Rotation: the right leg rotates to the right and vice versa, i.e., the right leg rotates clockwise as you look down on It

This might be a good time to stand up and move your legs around through these ranges of motion just to get a feel for the different movements in your body.

Movement in the Spine

The spine consists of five sections. The three upper sections—the cervical spine at the neck, the thoracic spine at the upper back, and the lumbar spine at the lower back—are made up of small bones called vertebrae, which are separated by fluid-filled vertebral disks. These cushionlike disks hold the vertebrae apart and allow them to move freely. The greatest range of motion in the spine is found in the cervical area, or neck, followed by the lumbar spine, or lower back. The range of motion in the cervical spine and the lumbar spine is ultimately restricted by the shape of the vertebrae themselves. The thoracic spine has less range of motion, not only because of the shape of its vertebrae but also because the ribs are attached to them. At the bottom of the spine are the sacrum and the coccyx. The five bones of the sacrum and the four bones of the coccyx are fused in adults and do not move separately.

The spine also moves in six different ways that are only slightly different from the movements of the femurs. They are shown below.

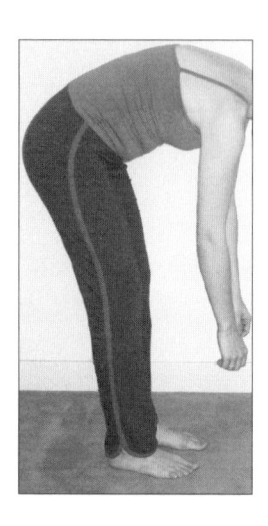

1. Flexion: the spine bends forward

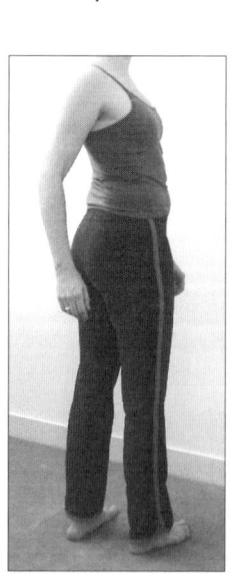

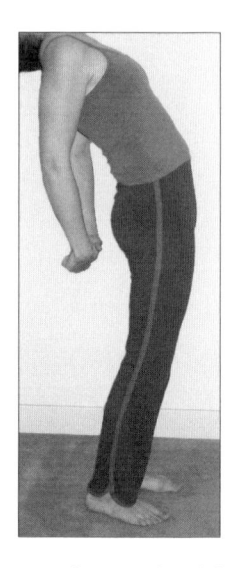

2. Extension: the spine bends backward

3. Rotation to the Right: the torso rotates to the right in relation to the pelvis (that's an easy one)

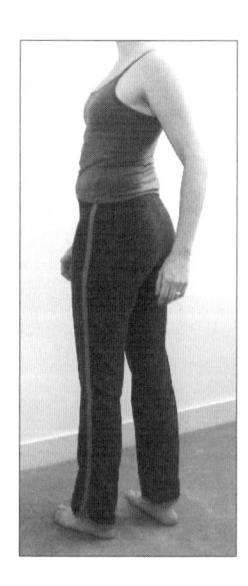

4. Rotation to the Left: the torso rotates to the left

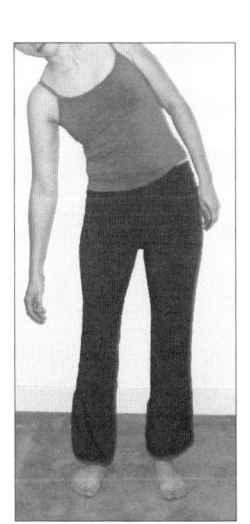

5. Lateral Flexion to the Right: the torso bends to the right side in relation to the pelvis

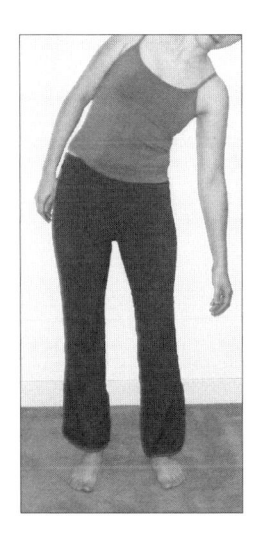

6. Lateral Flexion to the Left: the torso bends to the left in relation to the pelvis

Planning Your Yin Practice around Hip and Spine Movements

It is important to understand these hip and spine movements because one of the goals of Yin Yoga is to bring the joints between the knees and the navel safely and gently to their full range of motion in all the directions they move. All tissue in the body, whether it's muscle or connective tissue, tends to atrophy and lose its ability to function properly if it's not fully used. In taking these important joints to the extent of their range of motion, we can help keep the connective tissue healthy, the qi flowing, and the muscles flexible. Understanding how the body moves helps us know how to accomplish this goal and is important in planning and sequencing a practice. I always try to include postures that bring me into as many of these directions of movement as time and the way my body is feeling will allow. (When planning a practice with an eye to range of motion, see the table on page 108 called Spine and Hip Movement in Yin Postures to help you decide which postures to include.)

Yin Postures and Spine Movements

You may notice that the practice as I've presented it in this kit includes a number of spinal flexions (front bends), but only three spinal extensions (back bends). I try to always include at least two of the spinal extensions in any given practice sequence. I do this to balance the spinal flexions. In other words, I try to balance my forward bends with back bends. The only lateral flexions or side bends come in Half Butterfly and in Dragonfly when you lean more toward one side, rather than bending straight forward. I almost always include Half Butterfly in my practice because it provides some lateral flexion, yet it is also the easiest forward bend to do because the hamstring muscles are released on the bent-leg side. Spinal Twist is the only posture in this practice that rotates the spine, so I always include one twist to each side, even if I don't have time to hold them as long as the other postures.

Yin Postures and Hip Movements

That was a short, simple rundown of the postures and the way the spine moves, now let's look at how the hips move in different postures. You'll notice that in many of the postures the hip joint is flexed, externally rotated, and abducted (widened). As with back bends of the spine, there are only three postures that extend the femur in relation to the pelvis: Seal, Saddle, and Swan. It is as important to the hips as it is to the spine to include several of these extensions in any sequence. In our everyday movement, the femur is more often externally rotated and abducted than internally rotated and adducted. Notice that if you stand up and decide to walk to your right, you will most likely start with your right leg, externally rotating and abducting it, rather than starting with your left leg and internally rotating and adducting it. Shoelace is the only pose that strongly adducts (crosses) the femurs, so I practice it often. For some people, this strong adduction is very uncomfortable. If you are one of these people, I would suggest that you try doing Square Pose instead of Shoelace, which will usually provide a much milder and more pleasant but similar stretch. The only real internal rotation in the postures I've presented here come in Saddle, for people whose heals are outside their hips, and in Frog, for people who keep their feet wide apart. If neither of these things happen for you in your practice, please don't fret; you may still have a chance of living a happy life.

Using Range of Motion to Sequence Your Practice

By understanding that the body moves in certain specific ways, we can try to configure our practice so as to move it in as many ways as possible during any given sequence of poses. We can understand that by doing a posture that flexes our spine after doing one that extends it, we can bring balance to the practice and perhaps feel better in our bodies. Of course, everyone's body is different so please take this information as a guideline only and, as always, trust the wisdom of your own body and experience.

Let's look at the first one-hour practice that I lead on the CD. It begins with Half Butterfly because that is the easiest forward bend, especially when the body is cold. It also gives a nice abduction and external rotation to the bent leg. I include Seal next, a back bend to balance the forward bend. Frog is a nice counter pose to Seal and also abducts and for some people internally rotates the femurs. Shoelace (or Square Pose if Shoelace is too intense for you) follows, bringing the legs into adduction and external rotation. These poses are followed by the strongest back bend in the Yin practice, Saddle. Saddle is also an internal rotation for most people. Spinal Twist is a spinal rotation and leads smoothly into Resting Pose. This sequence is one that I practice often because it works for my body. I invite you to use the sequencing principles as I've explained them here to arrive at a series of postures that works best for you. The following table will help you remember how the spine and hips move in each posture.

SPINE AND HIP MOVEMENTS IN YIN POSTURES

Yin Postures	Movement of the Spine	Movement of the Hips
Forward Bend	Flexion	Flexion
Half Butterfly	Flexion Some Lateral Flexion	Flexion on Straight Leg Flexion, External Rotation, and Abduction on Bent Leg
Butterfly	Some Flexion	Some Flexion, External Rotation, and Abduction
Shoestring	Some Flexion	External Rotation, Adduction, and potentially Some Flexion
Seal	Extension	Extension
Saddle	Extension	Extension Internal Rotation when heels are outside hips
Square Pose	Flexion	External Rotation, Flexion, and Some Abduction
Frog	Some Flexion	Internal Rotation, Abduction, and Flexion if knees are forward
Dragonfly	Flexion Some Lateral Flexion by leaning toward one foot rather than toward the center	Abduction
Spinal Twist	Rotation	Flexion and Adduction of the bent leg
Swan	Extension	External Rotation, Abduction, and Flexion of the bent leg Extension of the straight leg
Sleeping Swan	Neutral	External Rotation, Abduction, and Flexion of the bent leg Straight leg is neutral
Resting Pose	Neutral	Flexion and Slight Internal Rotation
Final Relaxation	Neutral	Some Abduction

APPENDIX 1: SOME SAMPLE PRACTICES

These are only suggested practices. It is my hope that you will develop your own over time.

Two-Hour Practice
(18 postures at 5 minutes per posture with 1 minute of transition between postures, followed by a 10-minute meditation)

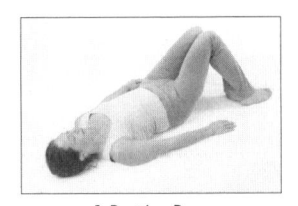

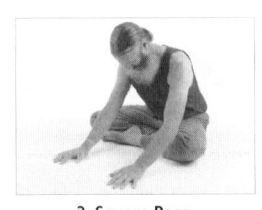

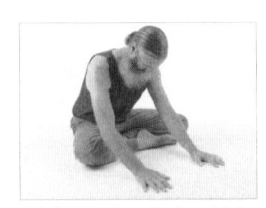

| 1. Resting Pose | 2. Square Pose | 3. Square Pose (other side) |

110 • APPENDIX 1

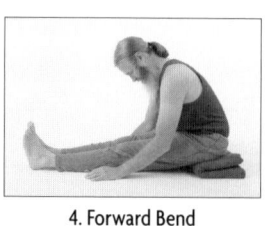

4. Forward Bend

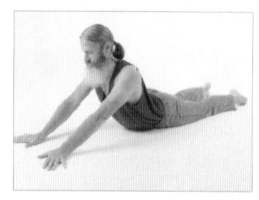

5. Seal

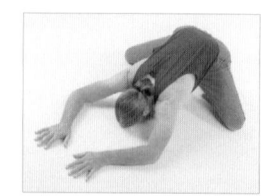

6. Frog

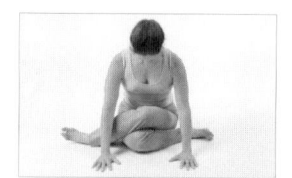

7. Shoelace

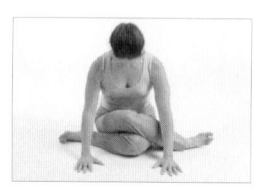

8. Shoelace (other side)

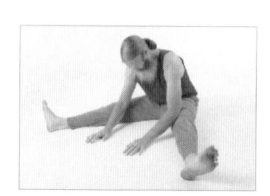

9. Dragonfly

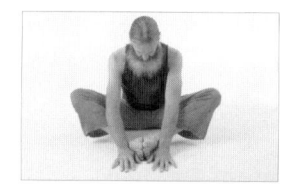

10. Butterfly

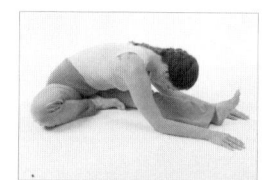

11. Half Butterfly

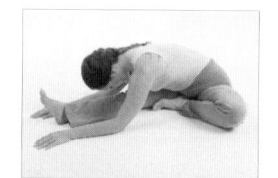

12. Half Butterfly (other side)

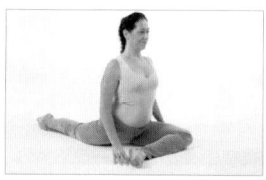

13. Swan to Sleeping Swan (5 minutes total)

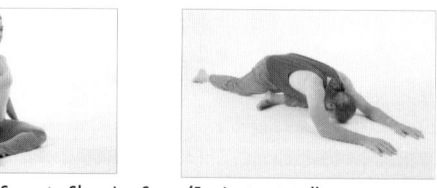

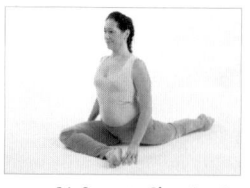

14. Swan to Sleeping Swan (other side) (5 minutes total)

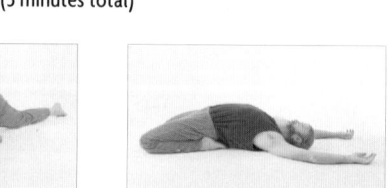

15. Saddle

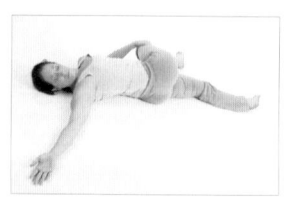

16. Spinal Twist

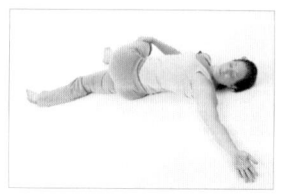

17. Spinal Twist (other side)

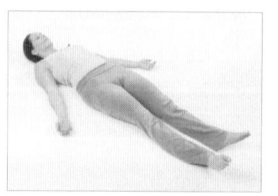

18. Final Relaxation

Some Sample Practices • 111

Ninety-Minute Practice

(15 postures at 5 minutes per posture with 1 minute of transition between postures)

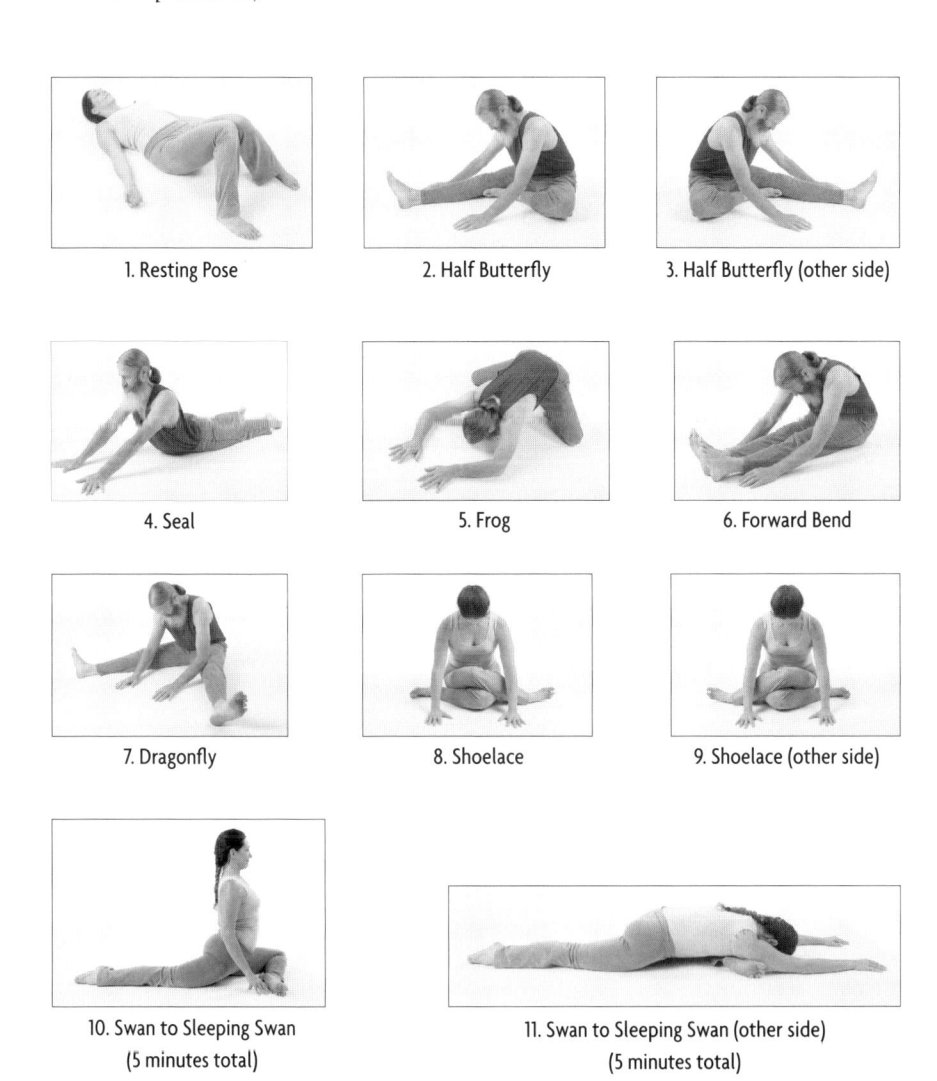

1. Resting Pose
2. Half Butterfly
3. Half Butterfly (other side)
4. Seal
5. Frog
6. Forward Bend
7. Dragonfly
8. Shoelace
9. Shoelace (other side)
10. Swan to Sleeping Swan (5 minutes total)
11. Swan to Sleeping Swan (other side) (5 minutes total)
12. Saddle

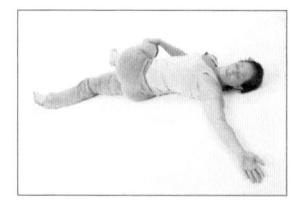

13. Spinal Twist

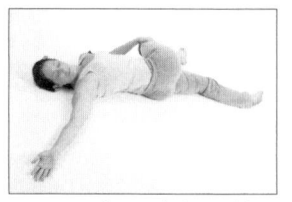

14. Spinal Twist (other side)

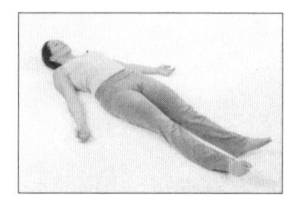

15. Final Relaxation

Some One-Hour Practices

One-Hour Practice A

(10 postures at 5 minutes per posture with 1 minute of transition between postures)

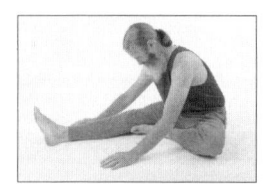

1. Half Butterfly

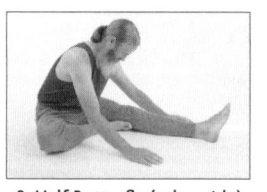

2. Half Butterfly (other side)

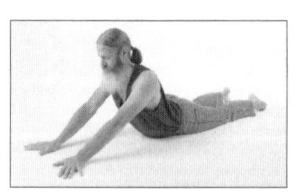

3. Seal

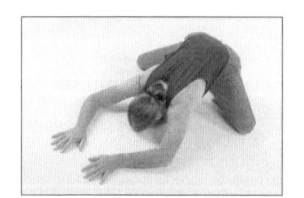

4. Frog

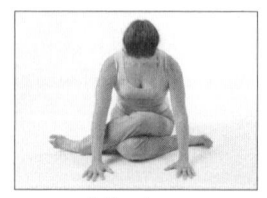

5. Shoelace

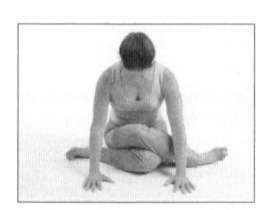

6. Shoelace (other side)

Some Sample Practices • 113

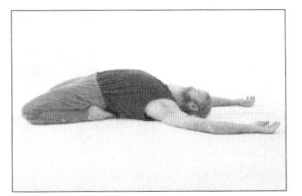

7. Saddle

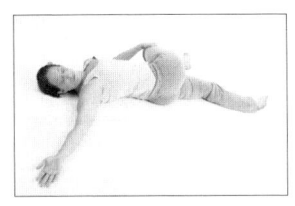

8. Spinal Twist

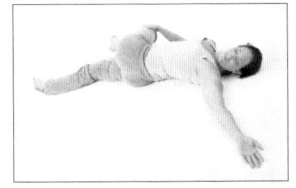

9. Spinal Twist (other side)

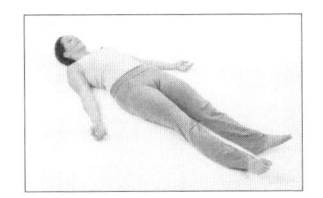

10. Final Relaxation

One-Hour Practice B

(10 postures at 5 minutes per posture with 1 minute of transition between postures)

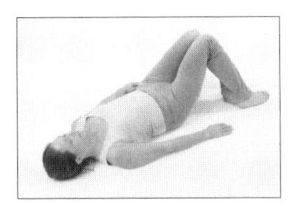

1. Resting Pose

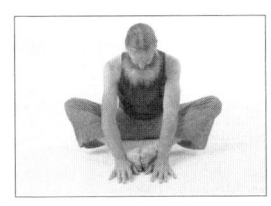

2. Butterfly

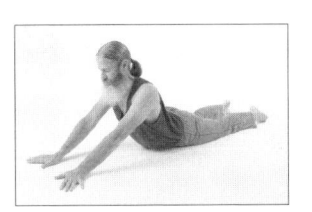

3. Seal

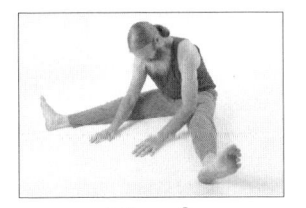

4. Dragonfly

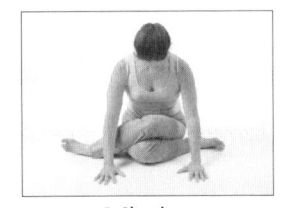

5. Shoelace

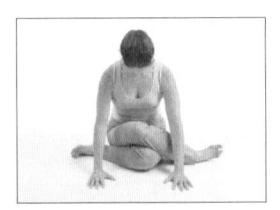

6. Shoelace (other side)

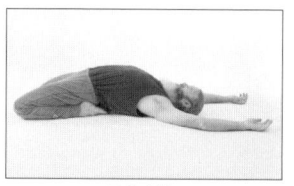

7. Saddle

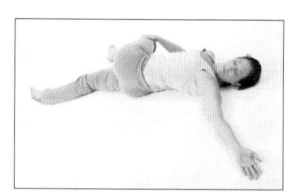

8. Spinal Twist

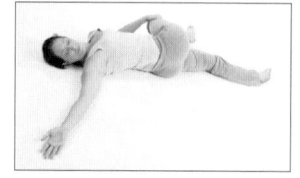

9. Spinal Twist (other side)

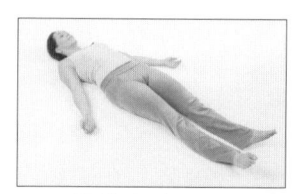

10. Final Relaxation

One-Hour Practice C

(9 postures at 5 minutes per postures with 1 minute of transition between postures, followed by a 5-minute meditation)

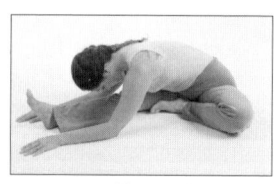

1. Half Butterfly

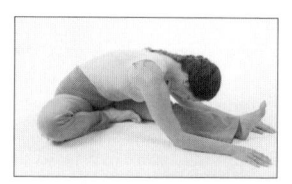

2. Half Butterfly (other side)

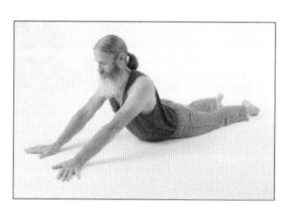

3. Seal

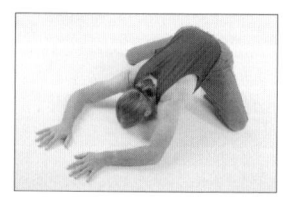

4. Frog

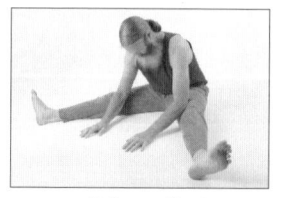

5. Dragonfly

SOME SAMPLE PRACTICES • 115

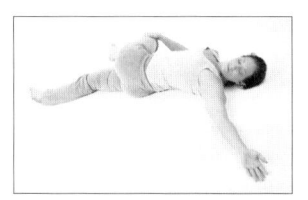

6. Spinal Twist

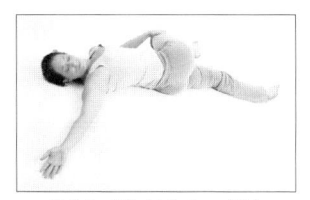

7. Spinal Twist (other side)

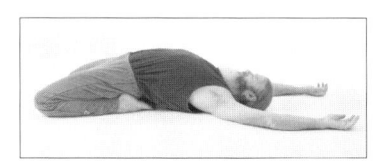

8. Saddle

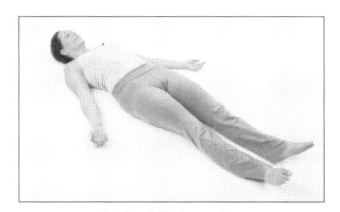

9. Final Relaxation

Some Thirty-Minute Practices

Thirty-Minute Practice A
(5 postures at 5 minutes per posture with 1 minute of transition between postures)

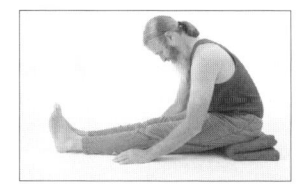

1. Forward Bend

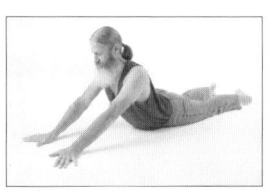

2. Seal

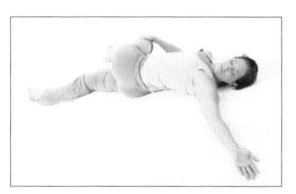

3. Spinal Twist

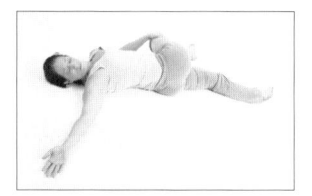

4. Spinal Twist (other side)

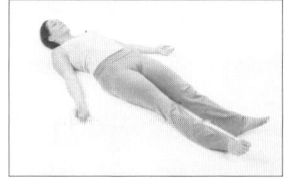

5. Final Relaxation

Thirty-Minute Practice B

(5 postures at 5 minutes per posture with 1 minute of transition between postures)

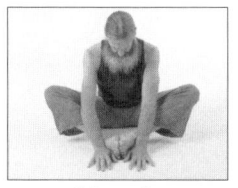

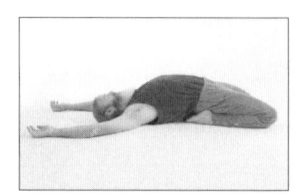

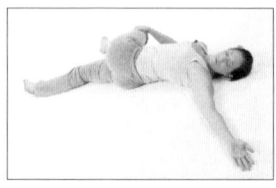

1. Butterfly
2. Saddle
3. Spinal Twist
4. Spinal Twist (other side)
5. Resting Pose

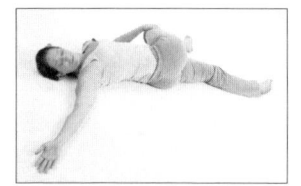

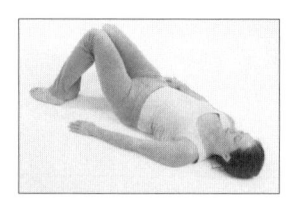

Thirty-Minute Practice C

(4 postures at 5 minutes per posture plus 2 postures at 3 minutes per posture with 1 minute of transition between postures)

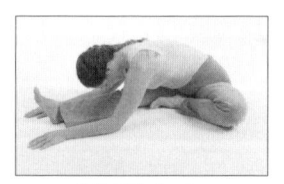

1. Half Butterfly
2. Half Butterfly (other side)
3. Seal
4. Frog
5. Spinal Twist (3 minutes)
6. Spinal Twist (3 minutes, other side)

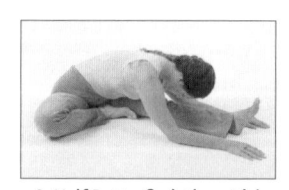

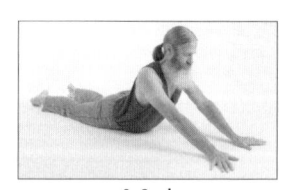

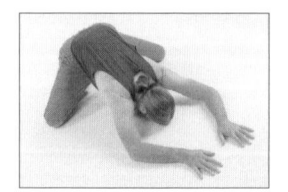

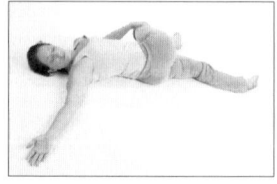

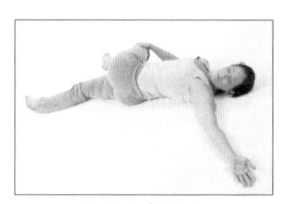

APPENDIX 2: PRACTICES FOR SPECIFIC ORGAN MERIDIANS

The practices in this appendix have been selected to stimulate specific organ meridians. If you have a specific physical or emotional challenge that you would like to work on, you can take a look at the Meridian Attributes table on page 18 to decide which of these practices would be most helpful. Alternatively, you could choose to do each of these practices on a regular rotation to bring attention to all of your meridians. These postures are not intended to cure specific ailments but to help bring attention and intention and to awaken our own healing energy.

One-Hour Practice Targeting the Stomach and Spleen Meridians

(10 postures at 5 minutes per posture with 1 minute of transition between postures)

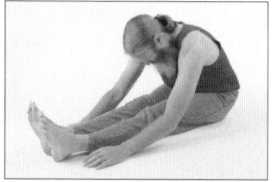

1. Forward Bend

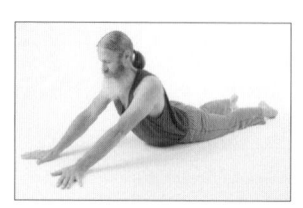

2. Seal

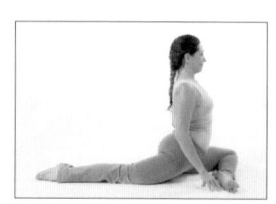

3. Swan

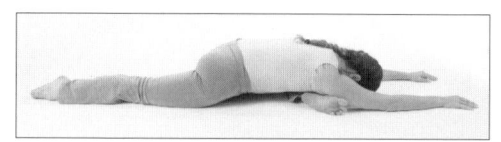

4. Sleeping Swan

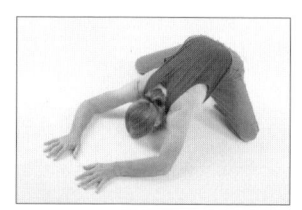

5. Frog

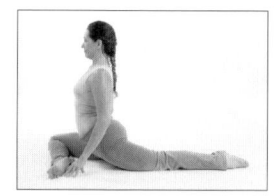

6. Swan (other side)

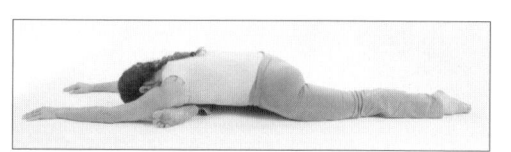

7. Sleeping Swan (other side)

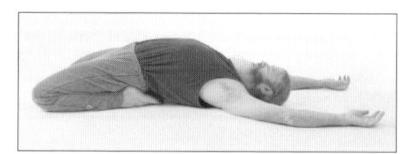

8. Saddle

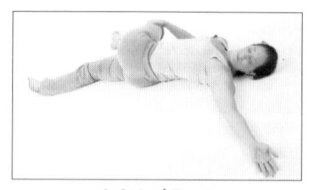

9. Spinal Twist
(switch sides halfway through)

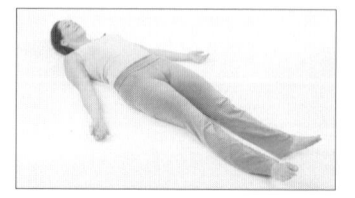

10. Final Relaxation

Practices for Specific Organ Meridians • 119

Ninety-Minute Practice Targeting the Liver and Gall Bladder Meridians

(15 postures at 5 minutes per posture with 1 minute of transition between postures)

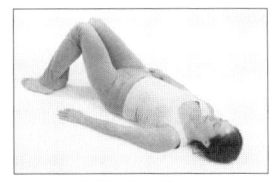

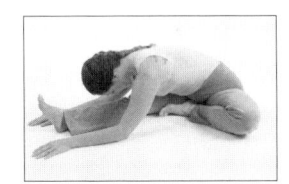

1. Resting Pose
2. Half Butterfly
3. Half Butterfly (other side)
4. Seal
5. Swan to Sleeping Swan (5 minutes total)
6. Swan to Sleeping Swan (other side) (5 minutes total)
7. Frog
8. Square Posture (reverse legs halfway through)
9. Dragonfly
10. Shoelace
11. Shoelace (other side)

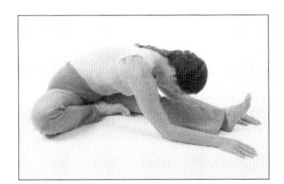

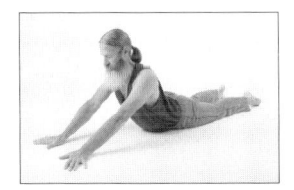

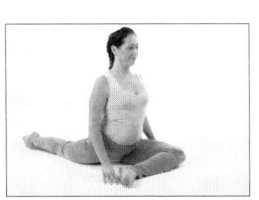

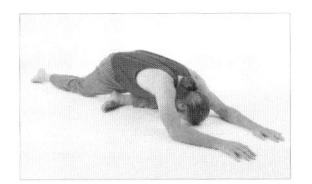

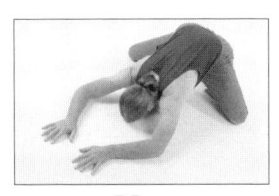

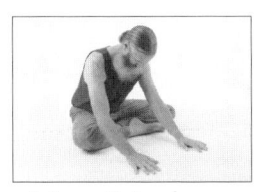

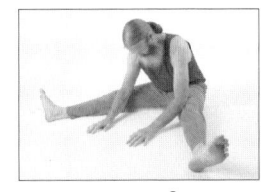

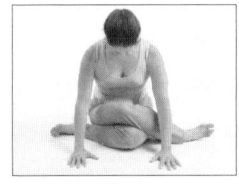

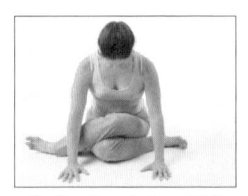

120 • APPENDIX 2

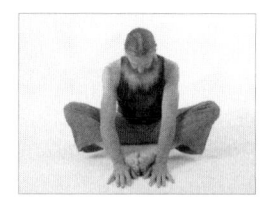

12. Butterfly

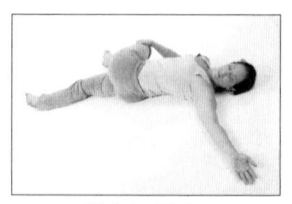

13. Spinal Twist

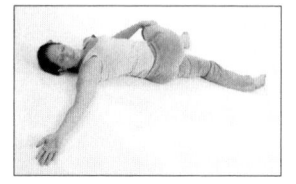

4. Spinal Twist (other side)

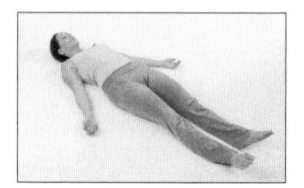

15. Final Relaxation

Ninety-Minute Practice Targeting the Kidney and Urinary Bladder Meridians

(15 postures at 5 minutes per posture with 1 minute of transition between postures)

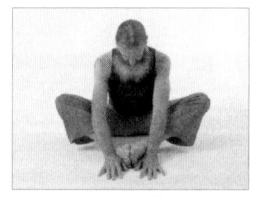

1. Butterfly

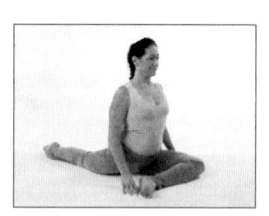

2. Swan to Sleeping Swan (5 minutes total)

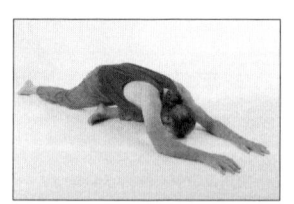

3. Swan to Sleeping Swan (other side) (5 minutes)

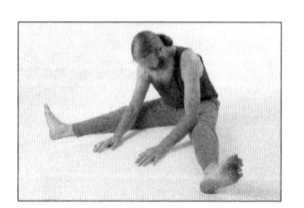

4. Dragonfly

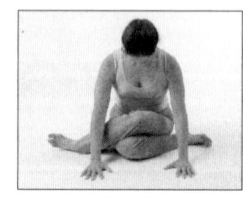

5. Shoelace

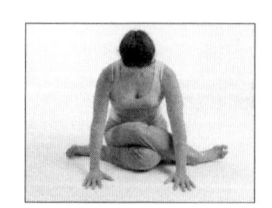

6. Shoelace (other side)

Practices for Specific Organ Meridians • 121

7. Frog

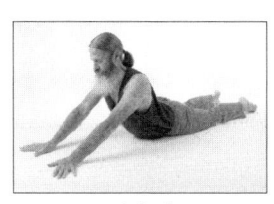

8. Seal

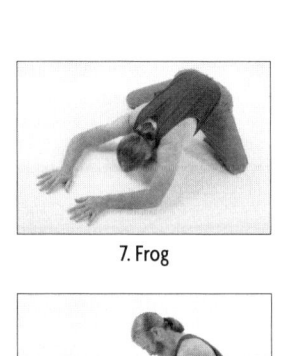

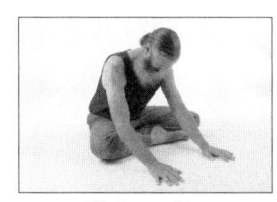

9. Forward Bend

10. Square Pose
(reverse legs halfway through)

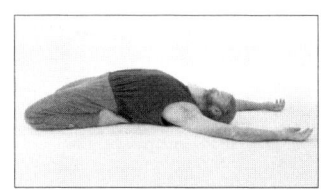

11. Saddle

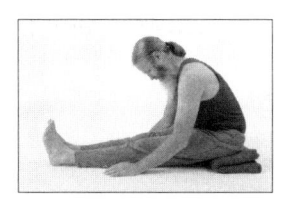

12. Forward Bend

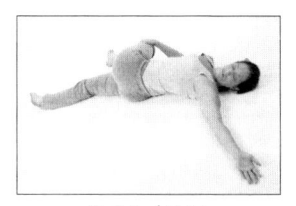

13. Spinal Twist

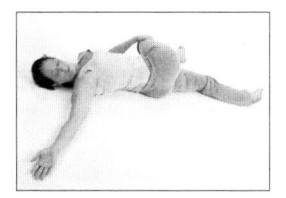

14. Spinal Twist (other side)

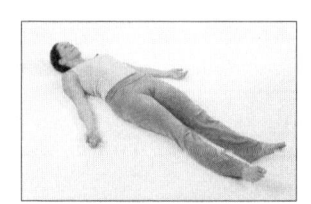

15. Final Relaxation

APPENDIX 3: USING ACUPRESSURE POINTS WHILE PRACTICING YIN YOGA

In my own practice, I've found that putting manual pressure on some of the classic acupuncture or acupressure points that can be reached while in Yin postures can increase the energetic effect of the posture. I suggest that once you have become comfortable with your Yin practice, you experiment with some of the acupressure points outlined here and see if using them as I've suggested adds to your experience.

I've chosen seven acupressure points on the feet and lower legs that I feel are beneficial. These points lie within reach while practicing many Yin poses. Not all points are reachable in all postures or by everyone. In some postures such as Frog, Seal, and Saddle, it is difficult to reach any of the points at all.

In Parts 1 and 2 we discussed the relationship of specific Yin postures to specific meridians. The best way to use acupressure in conjunction with your Yin practice is to stimulate acupressure points along a meridian that's already being stimulated by the posture you're holding. To refresh your memory of the meridians stimulated by each posture, see the table on page 30. You can also refer to the pages that describe each posture in Part 2.

First you need to locate the point along the meridian on either the left or right side, depending on which you can reach most easily. The table on the next page describes the location of each of the seven points. You'll also find drawings showing the point locations on page 125.

In the table, the directions for locating the points are given in "body units" relative to a specific spot on the body. One body unit is equal to the width of your thumb at its outermost joint. Three body units are equal to the width of your four fingers when held together. For instance, to find Spleen 6 as described in the table, you first locate the ankle bone on the inside of your foot, and then measure up the leg from the top of the ankle bone three body units (the width of all four fingers held together) and imagine a line around the inside of the leg at that height. If you follow that line to where it meets your shinbone, you will be near the point. In the beginning you may find it difficult to feel these points, but with a little practice it will become easier. Pay close attention as your fingers approach the spot. When you reach it, you will feel a slight indentation—a sort of vortex into which your fingers are drawn. As you push on the spot, it may feel more sensitive, even tender, compared to the surrounding area.

SOME ACUPRESSURE POINTS ACCESSIBLE IN YIN POSTURES

Acupressure Points	Location	Function
Kidney 3 (KD 3)	Between the ankle bone and the Achilles tendon on the inside (medial) side of the foot	Builds Kidney energy (Jing). Particularly important for men.
Urinary Bladder 60 (UB 60)	Between the ankle bone and the Achilles tendon on the outside (lateral) side of the foot. Opposite KD 3.	Relieves lower-back pain and tightness
Spleen 6 (SP 6)	Three body units above the upper edge of the inner (medial) ankle bone and just behind the shin bone (tibia)	Where the three Yin meridians (Liver, Kidney, and Spleen) meet. Builds Yin energy. Particularly important for women.
Gall Bladder 34 (GB 34)	On the outer (lateral) side of the leg just below the top of the fibula (the outside lower-leg bone), forward of the tendon but behind the muscle	The master point for releasing the tendons and ligaments
Stomach 36 (ST 36)	Three body units below the bottom edge of the knee cap (patella) and one body unit outside the shin bone (tibia), it can be most easily found with the knee slightly bent	A major energy point on the body. Helps build blood.
Liver 3 (LV3)	One body unit up from the edge of the webbing between the big toe and the second toe (the little piggy who went to market and the one who stayed home)	Moves stagnant Liver energy
Urinary Bladder 40 (UB 40)	Behind the knee, just outside (lateral to) the major tendon that runs on the inner (medial) side of the knee pit. There are two major tendons that you can feel behind the knee, UB 40 is outside the innermost, between it and the muscle outside it (lateral). You may find it easier to locate this point with your knee slightly bent.	A major point for affecting the lower back

Using Acupressure Points while Practicing Yin Yoga • 125

Once you locate a chosen point and are situated in your Yin posture, you can use your finger or thumb to apply pressure. How much pressure to use and how long to hold the pressure are very individual decisions, so listen to your own body. You may want to start by holding for a few seconds, gradually increasing up to the full time you're in the pose, or you may find that by putting pressure on the point for just a short time you'll bring awareness to the meridian and feel an immediate increase in the flow of qi. In the table, along with the point locations, I've listed the function of each point as it's classically seen in the practice of acupuncture.

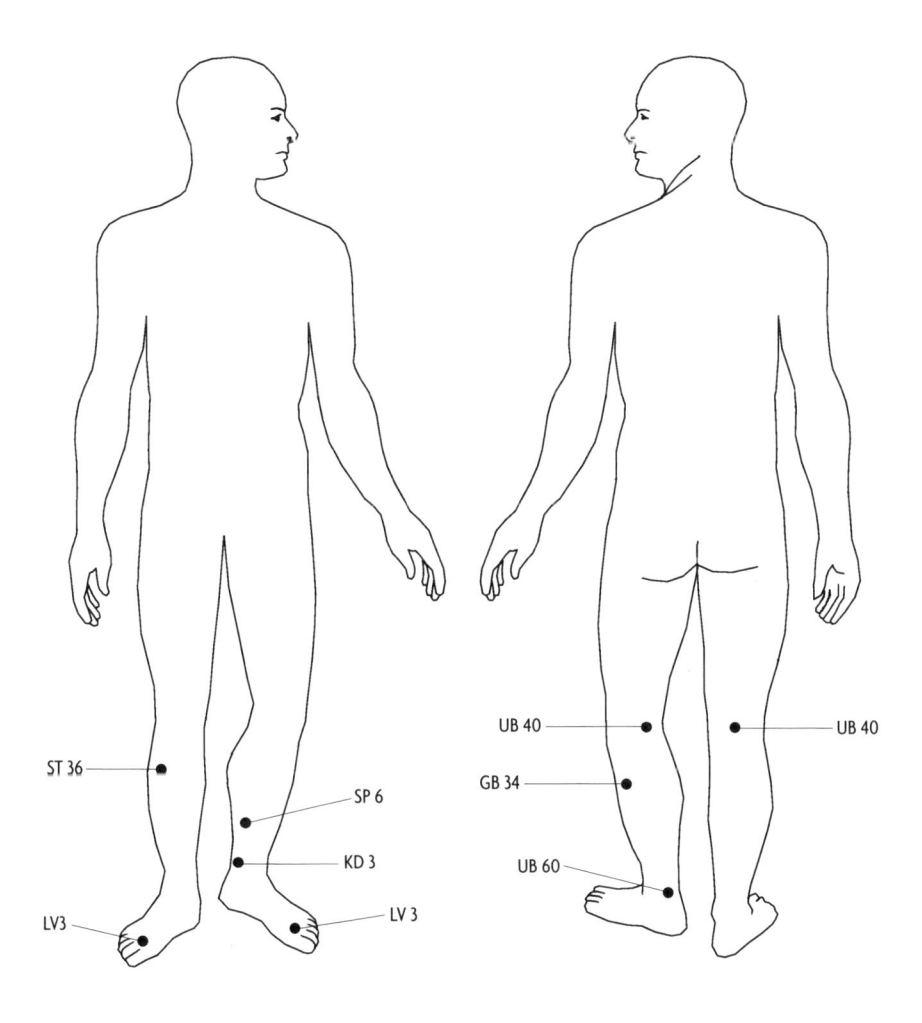

In acupuncture or acupressure, points are often used in combination in order to increase their effects. In Yin practice you can stimulate two points at the same time by reaching one point with one hand and one with the other or, in the case of Ki 3 and UB 60, by applying pressure with the thumb and finger of the same hand. In the table below, I've listed some combinations that you may want to try.

SOME EFFECTIVE COMBINATIONS OF ACUPRESSURE POINTS

Point Combinations	Positive Effects
GB 34+UB 40	Releases tendons and ligaments and relaxes lower back
UB 40+UB 60	Helps to release lower back
ST 36+SP 6	Helps fight fatigue and build energy
LV 3+SP 6	Moves stagnation out of liver Builds yin energy—especially useful for women
KD 3+SP 6	Builds energy—useful for men and women
UB 60+GB 34	Releases and relaxes lower back
KD 3+UB 60	Conveniently located to reach with one hand (you get 2 for 1) Acupuncturists sometimes put one needle all the way through both points Builds kidney energy and relaxes lower back

The final table in this appendix lists acupuncture points (and combinations of points) that I feel work well with specific postures. These points correspond with the meridians that are already being stimulated by the physical shape of each pose.

POTENTIAL POINTS AND COMBINATIONS FOR SPECIFIC POSTURES

Yin Postures*	Acupressure Points	Point Combinations
Half Butterfly	KD 3, UB 60, SP 6, GB 34, ST 36, LV 3, UB 40	GB 34+UB 40, UB 40+UB 60, ST 36+SP 6, LV 3+SP 6
Shoelace	KD 3, SP 6	KD 3+SP 6
Butterfly	KD 3, SP 6, LV 3	KD 3+SP 6
Forward Bend	KD 3, SP 6, UB 40, UB 60	KD 3+SP 6, UB 40+UB 60
Dragonfly	KD 3, UB 60, UB 40	Note: few people can reach KD 3 or UB 60 in Dragonfly but you can always practice with a friend
Square	KD 3, UB 60, GB 34	UB 60+GB 34
Swan	KD 3, UB 60	no obvious ones
Spinal Twist	GB 34	no obvious ones

*Note: I have not included any points for Seal, Saddle, Frog, Sleeping Swan, Resting Pose, or Final Relaxation as none can be easily reached in these postures.

The use of acupressure points is not necessary in any Yin practice, so don't be concerned if you don't feel any benefit in including them. As with all aspects of the practice I've presented, I invite you to take what makes sense for you and leave the rest.

RESOURCES

Books

Arrien, Angeles. *The Four-Fold Way: Walking the Paths of the Warrior, Teacher, Healer and Visionary.* San Francisco: HarperSan Francisco, 1993.

Avalon, Arthur. *The Serpent Power: The Secrets of Tantric and Shaktic Yoga.* New York: Dover Publications, 1974.

Bienfield, Harriet, L.Ac., and Erem Korngold, L.Ac., O.M.D. *Between Heaven and Earth: A Guide to Chinese Medicine.* New York, Ballantine Books, 1992.

Calais-Germain, Blandine. *Anatomy of Movement.* Seattle: Eastland Press, 1985.

Grilley, Paul. *Yin Yoga: Outline of a Quiet Practice.* Ashland, Ore.: White Cloud Press, 2002.

Hanh, Thich Nhat. *The Miracle of Mindfulness.* Boston: Beacon Press, 1987.

Jahnke, Roger, O.M.D. *The Healer Within.* San Francisco: HarperSan Francisco, 1999.

———. *The Healing Promise of Qi: Creating Extraordinary Wellness Through Qigong and Tai Chi.* New York: Contemporary Books, 2002. See also Dr. Jahnke's web site: www.feeltheqi.com.

Judith, Anodea, Ph.D. *Wheels of Life.* St. Paul, Minn.: Llewellyn Publications, 1987 and 1999.

Kaptchuk, Ted. *The Web That Has No Weaver: Understanding Chinese Medicine.* New York: McGraw Hill, 2000.

Kornfield, Jack. *The Art of Forgiveness, Lovingkindness, and Peace.* New York: Bantam Books, 2002.

Lao Tsu. *Tao Te Ching.* Gia-Fu Feng and Jane English, trans. New York: Vintage Books, 1997.

Motoyama, Hiroshi. *Awakening the Chakras and Emancipation.* Encinitas, Calif: Human Science Press, 2003.

Salzberg, Sharon. *Loving Kindness: The Revolutionary Art of Happiness.* Boston: Shambhala Publications, 1995.

Stapleton, Don, Ph.D. *Self-Awakening Yoga.* Rochester, Vt.: Healing Arts Press, 2004.

DVDs

Grilley, Paul. *Anatomy for Yoga* (DVD). San Francisco: Pranamaya, 2004.

———. *Yin Yoga: The Foundations of a Quiet Practice* (2-DVD set). San Francisco: Pranamaya, 2005.

Powers, Sarah. *Insight Yoga with Sarah Powers* (DVD). San Francisco: Pranamaya, 2005.

———. *Yin and Vinyasa Yoga with Sarah Powers* (DVD). Self-produced, 2002, available at www.sarahpowers.com.

Workshops

For information on upcoming Yin Yoga workshops or to schedule a workshop with Biff Mithoefer, please visit his Web site:

biffmithoeferyoga.com.

ACKNOWLEDGMENTS

I'm finding the writing of this part of the book to be very hard. When I try to express my deep gratitude for all the support I've received that has brought me to the completion of this project, I can't help but feel the inner connectedness of all beings. What being was not here with me every step of my life, every step of my yoga journey? I feel such gratitude to be a part of this thing we're all doing together, this search to "wash love clean of all its stories." I know that although it was the me that lives in this body who wrote this book, what wisdom it contains came from all the struggles of all beings on the path to find the way back to their own hearts.

There are, however, some people in my life to whom I want to express my gratitude directly:

- My family, Amy, Ben, and Peter
- My mother and father and my ancestors, whose wisdom and struggles I carry
- All my yoga teachers and all my students

Acknowledgments

Dr. Michael Mithoefer

Olivia Mithoefer

Dr. Norma Manrique

Roger Jahnke, O.M.D.

Dr. Experience Bryon

Dedier and Jose

Laurie, Ricci, and Jack

Angeles Arrien

Irene Cole, whose design made this project look possible

Rocki Pedersen for the wonderful photographs

Cheryl Moss for opening her studio, Goda Yoga, and posing for hours of pictures

Ann for teaching me and letting me teach with her

Jean for her support and for letting me use her picture on the cover

Ty Burhoe and Amy Ippoliti at Tala Records for the recording and friendship

Carlie and Kate for doing the practice

Laura, Jeanie, Susan, Peri, Rachel, Priscilla, Jon, Rob, Ehud, and all the other wonderful people at Inner Traditions International

And the Bodhisattvas, H. H. the Dalai Lama and Thich Nhat Hanh, who are here for us all.

BOOKS OF RELATED INTEREST

The Therapeutic Yoga Kit
Sixteen Postures for Self-Healing
through Quiet Yin Awareness
by Cheri Clampett and Biff Mithoefer

The Heart of Yoga
Developing a Personal Practice
by T. K. V. Desikachar

The Five Tibetans
Five Dynamic Exercises for Health,
Energy, and Personal Power
by Christopher S. Kilham

The Yoga-Sūtra of Patañjali
A New Translation and Commentary
by Georg Feuerstein, Ph.D.

Yoga Spandakarika
The Sacred Texts at the Origins of Tantra
by Daniel Odier

Pilates on the Ball
A Comprehensive Book and DVD Workout
by Colleen Craig

Natural Posture for Pain-Free Living
The Practice of Mindful Alignment
by Kathleen Porter

The New Rules of Posture
How to Sit, Stand, and Move in the Modern World
by Mary Bond

Inner Traditions • Bear & Company
P.O. Box 388
Rochester, VT 05767
1-800-246-8648
www.InnerTraditions.com

Or contact your local bookseller